The New Hypnosis
in Sex Therapy

The New Hypnosis in Sex Therapy

Cognitive-Behavioral Methods for Clinicians

Daniel L. Araoz, Ed.D.

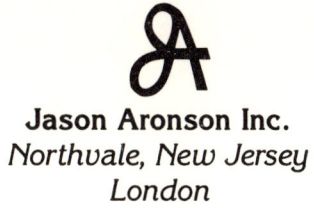

Jason Aronson Inc.
Northvale, New Jersey
London

THE MASTER WORK SERIES

First softcover edition 1998

Library of Congress Cataloging-in-Publication Data

Araoz, Daniel L., 1930–
    [Hypnosis and sex therapy]
    The new hypnosis in sex therapy : cognitive-behavioral methods for clinicians / Daniel L. Araoz. — 1st softcover ed.
       p.   cm. — (The Master work series)
    Originally published: New York : Brunner/Mazel, c1982.
    Includes bibliographical references and index.
    ISBN 0-7657-0137-5 (alk. paper)
    1. Sexual disorders—Treatment.   2. Hypnotism—Therapeutic use.
  3. Sex therapy. I. Title. II. Series.
    [DNLM: 1. Sex Disorders—therapy. 2. Hypnosis. Not Acquired]
  RC556.A68   1997
  616.6'906512—dc21
  DNLM/DLC
  for Library of Congress   97–34484

Printed in the United States of America on acid-free paper. For information and catalog write to Jason Aronson Inc., 230 Livingston Street, Northvale, New Jersey 07647-1731. Or visit our website: http://www.aronson.com

To Kaylee,
sunshine, laughter, innocence,
and joy in my life

Contents

Foreword

This book is the work of a professional who is dedicated to his work, devoted to his clients, diligent and disciplined in his approach, and demanding when looking for his clients' cooperation and success orientation.

Daniel Araoz here provides us with a wealth of hypnotherapeutic techniques, presented in the context of sex therapy. His New Hypnosis concept, emanating from years of clinical experience, may inspire theoretical controversy. Araoz's outlook on sex is relaxed and realistic. He does away with Herculean myths as well as with performance pressure. Standards are individualized and success is measured against personal interest, goals, and preference.

In his book, Araoz has pulled together a superb collection of techniques which is a source of inspiration to the beginning sex-hypnotherapist and is strongly recommended to all neophytes in psychotherapy. It is of equal importance as an anthology of techniques for accomplished sex hypnotherapists, encouraging them to use techniques which were never integrated into their routine armamentarium.

Questions about the essence of hypnosis have been asked again and again and have been answered over and over, yet never so that an agreement by all experts in hypnosis could be reached. Initially, the term "hypnosis" ("sleep" in Greek) was applied to phenomena believed to be artificial sleep. But others explained the same phenomena differently, namely as a state of hypersuggestibility, or as a pathological state, hysterical or dissociative in nature. Phenomenological and descriptive inquiries have referred to hypnosis as a trance state, an altered state of consciousness, a state of relaxation, a state of receptivity. Specific theories have explicated hypnotic phenomena on grounds of conditioning, concentration, regression to the womb, atavistic regression, role-playing, suggestion, dissociation, and self-organization. Physiological concomitants of hypnotic states have been recorded as specific brainwave activity, parasympathetic arousal, and nondominant brain hemisphere activation.

The depth of hypnosis has also been an issue; the question has been raised: Compared to non-hypnotic states, does hypnosis bring about a qualitative difference, or is it simply a matter of a quantitative more? Is whatever makes up the hypnotic state already present in our normal everyday experience? And is it merely due to an increase or expansion of this essence of hypnosis that labels like a mild, a medium, and a deep state of hypnosis became relevant indicators of intensity degrees? Is the difference in observable phenomena the symptomatic by-product of varied levels of hypnotic involvement? Or do the different symptoms originate from qualitatively different states?

Daniel Aaroz answers these questions in his own way. While taking note of the historical developments in the hypnosis field, he largely bypasses theoretical argumentation and pragmatically redefines hypnosis to suit his clinical, experiential model. In distinction from traditional hypnosis he calls it The New Hypnosis.

The New Hypnosis is defined as the mental state in which experiential thinking occurs while functioning of the logical, critical faculties is suspended. This experiential thinking occurs deliberately or spontaneously. It appears as daydreaming, fantasizing, imagining, connecting to unconscious realities while dissociating from the actual surrounding world, as viewing and reliving old memories, as age regression or progression, and so forth. It can involve purposeful goal-directed intervention in unconscious processes and programming or it can take the form of a spontaneous, free-floating experience connecting one to inner riches and creative powers. In a therapeutic situation, trust is emphasized as a major force in the relationship between client and therapist, but also as a factor in self-hypnosis where the necessary "letting go" demands trusting one's inner constructive forces.

The essence of The New Hypnosis is more definitely defined by what is excluded from it, than by what it includes. Excluded is logical, critical thinking, which is the antithesis of The New Hypnosis. Much of what is included in The New Hypnosis may coincide with the familiar, traditional views of hypnosis, but then, again, in logical consequence of the theory, a phenomenon as simple and common as daydreaming is now considered to be hypnosis. The "depth" of hypnosis is re-termed "height" of hypnosis, marking on a quantitative continuum the side of increased involvement.

More specifically defined is Araoz's concept of negative self-hypnosis (NSH), which he initially proposed in 1979. His formulation builds on empirical grounds. Negative self-hypnosis grows out of negative self-perceptions. Our noncritical processing activates subconscious mechanisms, reinforcing the bias through imagery, and finally, in the form of negative affirmation, leads to powerful autosuggestions. Inasmuch as NSH is emotionally determined and does not result from critical, logical thinking, Araoz categorizes it as hypnosis. NSH is rooted in the personal, perceptual filtering system with which phenomenologists are concerned in their understanding of the individual worlds people live in. We all operate from and within our own "my world" experience, as I like to call it. Torbjörn Stockfeldt (1973) names our biased world experience the "individual reality." He suggests that our world experience resulting from this individualized assimilation and perception process amounts to a hypnotic state. The challenging new question he sees emerging is: "When are we not hypnotized?" Thus, compared to Stockfeldt's position, Araoz's stance is less extreme.

Araoz is not alone in finding hypnosis in subliminal, in normal, ordinary, as well as in extraordinary states. Goba's thinking (1981) may in some respects be most akin to his. Yet he sees himself more directly connected to the positions held by Barber, Diamond, De Stefano and Katz, and many of the other thinkers who have, albeit in diverse directions, shared in demythologizing hypnosis, exploring its essence from their own perspectives.

When putting the search for the essence of hypnosis in historical perspectives, an interesting fact emerges. The realm of hypnosis expands and shrinks in direct proportion to the term's desirability, status and appeal. When the hypnosis halo effect is great and provides a favorable therapeutic impact on the client, then much of what is done becomes hypnosis. When, however, the halo gets tarnished and critical, contemporary thinking categorizes it as outdated quackery, then the hypnosis concept shrinks and even the use of those techniques originally and traditionally related to hypnosis are disclaimed as constituting practice of hypnosis.

Two examples shall illustrate this point. They involve Paul Hartenberg and Emile Coué. Hartenberg denied, in an essay published in 1898, that he was practicing hypnosis. He was treating his patients with artificial sleep (sommeil provoqué) and suggestion and insisted that hypnotism explained as a function of provoked sleep is nothing but an illusion. And Coué (1923) who, in a monotonous voice, led patients into a light state of "somnolence" to be more effective with his suggestions, declared: "I do not use hypnotism, nothing would be more untrue or more absurd" (p. 146).

Today, hypnosis—powerful, reputable, and even "medically approved"—attracts patients and therapists alike. Many people have opinions about hypnosis. Some perceive hypnosis as a normal state, some as a therapeutic tool, even as a cure-all, some as a dangerous weapon, and others as a profitable trick. Interest groups have become involved in regulatory issues. Laws have been passed and rules made to govern the practice of hypnosis. However, in the absence of a valid definition of hypnosis, law enforcement can become a difficult task. The only safely enforceable issue may be the legitimate or unauthorized use of the word "hypnosis." And just while the issue of importance of semantics and conceptualization is becoming an urgent focus point, the hypnosis avant-garde moves on, spreading the word that almost anything may be hypnosis and that hypnotic states are normal states.

This brings us back to Daniel Araoz. Is his hypnosis theory revolutionary? Is it inflationary? With others in the same tradition, what has he done by declaring normal states to be hypnotic? Has he desecrated our holy cow and let it out? Or was the holy cow already gone and is he simply, in its aftermath, once more clearly establishing that the word "hypnosis" embraces almost everything and that hypnosis does not work as mystery and magic. Yet he will not deny that the appeal, magic and the mystery still invested in the word "hypnosis" support the clients' confidence and courage to learn to take over their conscious and unconscious forces in order to set themselves free.

In the final analysis, what is the major contribution of this book on *Hypnosis and Sex Therapy?* Is it that Daniel Araoz shares his views, skills, and techniques as a sex therapist? Or is it that he provides us grounds for controversy as an expert in hypnosis? He gives us both. Sharing is the author's gift right now. Controversy, meaning movement, life, development, and growth, is his gift that reaches into the future.

Erika Wick, Ph.D.
Professor of Psychology,
St. John's University,
New York, N.Y.

REFERENCES

COUÈ, E. *My Method, Including American Impressions.* London, 1923.

GOBA, H. Know and use the power of your thoughts. *Reference Manual for Patients,* Calgary, Canada, 1981.

HARTENBERG, P. Essai d'une psychologie de la suggestion. *Revue de Psychologie Clinique et Thérapeutique.* 1898, 2, 264-278.

STOCKFELDT, T. When are we not hypnotized? In L. E. Unestahl (Ed.), *Hypnosis in the Seventies.* (6th Intl. Congress for Hypnosis, Uppsala 1973), Sweden: Veje Förlag Örebro, 1975.

Preface to the Softcover Edition

Since it first appeared, this book has been translated into Italian (1984), French (1994), and Spanish (1996), a fact indicating the continuing interest in the use of hypnosis for sexual dysfunctions. Because human sexual behavior is highly subjective—beliefs, values, expectations, and the like—the *systemic-cognitive-psychodynamic* perspective of this book remains the most comprehensive and effective method of treatment. One of my later books, *The New Hypnosis* (1985 and 1995), also published by Jason Aronson, expands the method used here to therapy with individuals and families.

The clinician who is not a specialist in sex therapy still needs a concrete perspective and practical techniques to help patients with the common psychogenic sexual dysfunctions that will, inevitably, be part of the therapeutic repertoire and that often affect the patient's self image, confidence, and esteem; interpersonal relationships; and even work (see Muchinsky 1993). *The New Hypnosis in Sex Therapy*, with the three theoretical elements just mentioned, becomes a method that can fit into any therapeutic modality, except the purely behavioristic, Skinnerian one. All therapists can enrich their treatment of sexual dysfunctions by adding to their practice the principles and techniques of this book.

Before proceeding with the theory that justifies and validates sex hypnotherapy, another important aspect for clinical sex therapy is in order. The *DSM-IV* muddles the difference between sexual dysfunction and disorder, upgrading highly treatable (see Seligman 1993), inevitable problems of the human condition to the rank of "mental disorders." Can we even consider generally the paraphilias as mental disorders, when the symptoms occur at the level of fantasy and desire, not of behavior? A serious difficulty lies in the lack of agreement about definitions among those who refuse to take the psychiatry manual as the infallible higher authority on mental disorders. Regardless of definitions, most psychogenic sexual dysfunctions are not to be listed in a manual of mental disorders. In the sexual area, *acedia*, described by Seligman as "the torpor of the soul, the indifference that creeps up on us as we age and grow accustomed to those we love [and] poisons so much of our life" (p. 173), is closely related to *abulia* in this book, and responds well to the treatment used for the latter. Though concerns about the AIDS epidemic nowadays rightly dominate the field of human sexuality, AIDS is beyond the scope of this book, limited, as it is, to the sexual dysfunctions that, in most cases, are not necessary indications of mental disorders. On the other hand, to engage in careless, unsafe sex is one of the clear indications of serious mental disorders, as are sexual activity with children, rape, and other such behaviors.

The classic 700-plus page-long text on human sexuality by Masters, Johnson, and Kolodny (1996) devotes only one out of twenty-five chapters to sexual dysfunctions and therapy. The chapter ends with a section on preventing sexual dysfunctions, a sober admonition not to overreact to them and to view sex as a joyful opportunity for self growth, rather than as a job to be performed. Once organic factors have been excluded, therapists, too, must be careful not to rush to interpret ordinary sexual difficulties as pathology and to avoid looking for more complicated reasons for the dysfunction than the psychosocial factors responsible for it. These factors may be developmental, like a traumatic first sexual experience or rigid religious beliefs; personal shortcomings, like sexual ignorance or naivete; and problems in interpersonal relations or, more specifically, with a particular partner. Also, assumptions by therapists that sexual dysfunctions are often, if not always, indications of early sexual abuse are likewise a disservice to effective therapy. Being vigilant for that possibility is very different than the currently popular quasi-conviction on the part of the therapist regarding the nearly universal presence of sexual abuse. The exploration techniques described in the book are useful for eliciting information that might have been repressed, always keeping in mind Spanos' (1996) cautions about unwittingly creating false memories.

To return to the theoretical components of this approach, the *cognitive* element is related to the ultimate goal of sex hypnotherapy. This is not merely to overcome the dysfunction but to help the couple enrich their future sexual experiences. In other words, the hope is that after therapy the couple will not merely go back to where they were before the sexual dysfunction started, but will have a more satisfying, more exciting, and fuller sexual exchange than ever before. For this, sex hypnotherapy, unlike more traditional methods, places special emphasis on *negative self-hypnosis* or what people "say to themselves" about their sexual pleasure and activities, their sexual fantasies, their bodies, and their partners, teaching them to make their self-talk (with all the images and feelings it generates) more effective for the attainment of their goals, in sex as well as in every other aspect of their lives. Because hypnosis is always self-hypnosis, this approach stresses the patient's need to practice in private the self-hypnotic techniques that were learned during the therapy sessions. The mind practice between therapy sessions is an essential component of this type of sex hypnotherapy. The purpose of the self-help injunction is twofold: to reinforce the benefits of the face-to-face session and to structure sex hypnotherapy as a program requiring committed work on the part of patients. Zilbergeld's (1992) self-help book is a useful complement to the cognitive aspect of sex hypnotherapy.

Because of the very nature of sexual behavior, which is cooperative, interdependent as well as mutually understanding, and respectful, sex hypnotherapy is also *systemic*. It is lastingly effective when it is approached this way, as the Masters and Johnson model taught us, and continues to be so in spite of criticism. Moreover, in this way of thinking we now include other systems besides the immediate, sex partner system, such as the subsystems of work, subculture, religious affiliation, and others that often affect one's attitudes toward sexual thinking and conduct.

Finally, the *psychodynamic*, highly subjective, and idiosyncratic elements present in all human behavior, including sexual, are ignored only to the detriment of an effective solution to sexual dysfunctions. It is curious that *cognitive* has been linked to behavior therapy and not emphasized enough in psychodynamic therapy when, in practice, many cognitive factors are affected directly by the psychodynamics of the individual, especially in a sexual relation.

Many years of experience have convinced me that the *hidden symptom* is still crucial to treating any sexual dysfunction. And because the hidden symptom is closely related to negative self-hypnosis, no progress can be expected without careful attention to the views patients have of their symptoms. The change of perception, belief, and interpretation regarding one's sexual problem is a form of experiential, rather than intellectual, reframing that, thanks to hypnosis, is accomplished quicker than through argument or didactic means and that operates at deep levels of one's being.

The way of thinking about symptoms, therapy, and hypnosis, of sexual dysfunctions and behavior in general, may demand unusual open-mindedness and mental flexibility on the part of the reader. Many letters received and numerous invitations to present this technique to professional audiences convince me that a large number of psychotherapists and specialists in sexual dysfunctions, from countries of the four different languages in which this book exists, have found the approach presented in *The New Hypnosis in Sex Therapy* useful for their practice, effective, and lasting in its results.

I am honored to have been invited to republish this book in the Master Work Series of Jason Aronson Inc.

Daniel L. Araoz, Ed.D.

REFERENCES

AMERICAN PSYCHIATRIC ASSOCIATION (1994). *Diagnostic and Statistical Manual of Mental Disorders, Fourth Edition.* Washington, DC: American Psychiatric Association.

ARAOZ, D. L. (1985). *The New Hypnosis: Techniques in Brief Individual and Family Psychotherapy.* Northvale, NJ: Jason Aronson, 1995.

MASTERS, W. H., JOHNSON, V. E., AND KOLODNY, R. C. (1996). *Human Sexuality, Fifth Edition.* New York: HarperCollins.

MUCHINSKY, P. (1993). Psychology Applied to Work. Pacific Grove, CA: Brooks/Cole.

SELIGMAN, M. E. P. (1993). *What You Can Change . . . and What You Can't.* New York: Fawcett Columbine.

SPANOS, N. P. (1996). *Multiple Identities and False Memories: A Sociocognitive Perspective.* Washington, DC: American Psychological Association.

ZILBERGELD, B. (1992). *The New Male Sexuality: The Truth about Men, Sex and Pleasure.* New York: Bantam.

Introduction

Applications of hypnosis to the treatment of sexual dysfunctions have been published sporadically, at least in the last three decades, as a perusal of the *International Journal of Clinical and Experimental Hypnosis* shows. Many clinicians have found hypnosis beneficial in dealing with sexual problems, both behaviorally and psychodynamically. However, very few sex therapists have made reference to hypnosis as such in their work. Even *The Journal of Sex Research,* founded by the late Dr. Hugo Beigel, one of the pioneers in the use of hypnosis in sex therapy, published only a handful of articles on hypnosis over a 17-year period.

One of the reasons for the scarce use of hypnosis in sex therapy in particular and in psychotherapy in general lies in the misconceptions about hypnosis which even now are rampant among clinicians. Another reason is that many practitioners who have taken a two- or three-day workshop on hypnosis go back to their practices and try the new-learned technique—only to discover that it isn't as easy as it sounded and looked during the workshop. Since most of these workshops have no follow-up, a large percentage of these students revert back to their familiar clinical modes and abandon hypnosis.

This book aims to offer the clinician a comprehensive understanding of the use of hypnosis in sex therapy. Thus, I have organized it in two parts: *Foundations* and *Applications.* From the outset, it must be stressed that hypnosis is used here in the modern way, namely, placing under the term any mental activity which is more experiential than critical, more subjective than outer-reality-oriented, more primary-process than secondary-process thinking, more right hemispheric than left hemispheric. The ritual of inducing hypnosis, the degree of hypnotizability, and the depth of the hypnotic experience are not stressed as much in modern hypnosis as in classical hypnosis. The new hypnosis stresses the cognitive skills involved in experiencing hypnosis, the work of the subject in activating new cognitive skills, the choice made by the subject to experience a change in consciousness. The validation of the cognitive-skills model of hypnosis comes from the research of Barber (1976) and his collaborators and from the work of other investigators, including Diamond (1977) and Katz (1979), who have expanded on the original ideas of Barber, as Chapter One will explain.

In sex therapy there is a new awareness of the importance of *cognitions* in normal sexual functioning. What happens inside the person —the mind activity, to use Barbara Brown's (1980) expression—is the key to what the person experiences in his/her sexual behavior. But the problem is that most people who engage in negativistic "thinking" do so non-consciously. Brown's sober considerations on "mind-apart-from-brain," coming as they do from a respected scientific researcher on the brain, make us question the thoroughness of the traditional approach to sex therapy. Her careful analysis of "mind" seems to justify our statement that sex is an attitude of mind.

Hypnosis is a proven tool or technique for reaching the non-conscious mind (Fromm et al., 1970) and because of its nature it is a highly effective approach to sex therapy. The person suffering from psychogenic sexual dysfunctions is most frequently engaged in what I call *negative self-hypnosis,* the non-conscious process by which negative affirmations or self-talk and defeatist mental images are either passively accepted or actively encouraged. This process is the "turn-off" mechanism Kaplan (1979) mentions in reference to inhibited sexual desire.

If negative self-hypnosis becomes a psychic antibody for sexual functioning, "positive" hypnosis, especially self-hypnosis, makes "regression in the service of pleasure," as Kaplan genially describes it, possible. Indeed, Mosher (1980) has made it clear that one of the natural elements of healthy sex is detachment from the generalized reality orientation of wakefulness, so that one can immerse oneself completely in the sexual experience. Hypnosis is also described in terms of dissociation from the external reality.

Part II of the book takes a closer look at both general and specific techniques and methods for the use of hypnosis in sex therapy. The clinical principles underlying the techniques are stressed, so that the mature clinician will be able to use the techniques flexibly and devise new ones according to the needs of his/her clientele.

My interest in writing this book is to help integrate the two fields of hypnosis and sex therapy, since the existing material is too scattered and disorganized to be of help for the busy practitioner. Lazarus (1976) claimed that much therapy is a waste of time. I believe that this statement becomes absolutely true if the therapist is not aware of the negative cognitive processes interfering with therapy and is not equipped with the clinical tools to combat negative self-hypnosis.

Were the book a superficial listing of practical hypnotic techniques to be used in sex therapy, its name would have been *Hypnosis in Sex Therapy*. However, since my intention is to present uses of hypnosis in sex therapy after having evaluated the evidence for the natural integration of both fields and after theorizing about such integration, its name is *Hypnosis* and *Sex Therapy*.

The book is written, primarily, for the sex therapist who intends to enrich his/her work with the use of hypnosis. But secondarily, it is also intended for the clinician who has already mastered hypnosis as a clinical tool and wants to focus more specifically on its application to sexual dysfunctions. I am, therefore, assuming that the reader is not a tyro in either field. *

I wish I could say truly that this book is the definitive work on hypnosis and sex therapy. Alas, no! Its contribution is, rather, in attempting to start an integration of the two fields after all these years in which each has developed so much useful information for the other. My hope

---

A book like this is helpful as a reference after one has had sufficient training in hypnosis to feel comfortable with its use in general. For the best professional training available, the two interprofessional organizations are The American Society of Clinical Hypnosis (2250 East Devon Ave., Des Plains, IL 60018) and The Society for Clinical and Experimental Hypnosis (129-A Kings Park Drive, Liverpool, NY 13088). Both have local chapters and training programs for beginners as well as for advanced students.

is that some of my ideas, controversial at times, will kindle renewed interest, discussion, and exchange among professionals in both fields.

Before beginning, I want to stress that this book applies to homosexual behavior as well as to heterosexuality, to "traditional" sex as well as to the myriad forms of unconventional sex. I consider any form of sexual behavior wholesome, beautiful, and enriching *as long as the participants are free, act by mutual accord and with mutual respect and sensitivity, and are ready to assume responsibility for their actions.* Spouses will be mentioned frequently. However, the principles and techniques expounded in this book have also been used successfully with nontraditional sexual partners.

The book is the result of many hours doing sex hypnotherapy and of many workshops teaching this approach both at the Annual Workshops of the American Society of Clinical Hypnosis and for the American Institute for Psychotherapy and Psychoanalysis in New York. To every one of the clients and colleagues who gave me so much while I was giving to them, I owe my deepest gratitude.

The New Hypnosis
in Sex Therapy

Part I

The Foundations

It was Agent 007 who believed that "you only live twice, once in your mind and once in your life." It was Virgil, before him, who stated: "They change their being, because they see themselves changing their being." Ellis (Ellis and Harper, 1961) has maintained since the beginnings of Rational Emotive Therapy that we are what we think. Later, Shorr (1974, 1977), among others, developed techniques to use our mental images for therapeutic purposes, basing his method on the evidence (Singer and McCraven, 1961) that 96 percent of people use mental images, imagination or fantasy regularly. This evidence comes from serious research (Singer, 1975, 1979) which found that the exception is *not* to imagine, that what we call *thinking* is indeed a mental reproduction of external reality by the use of our internal senses, which mirror the basic five receptive systems by which we interact with the external world.

Following the thinking of Ahsen (1979), Sheehan (1979) and many others, I take imagery in the broad sense of inner representational systems of our experience; I do not limit mental images to visual or pictorial representations, but include under the mental-image concept auditory, gustatory, olfactory and kinesthetic representations as well. This view is shared by many prominent figures in the fields of psychotherapy (e.g., Lazarus, 1977) and of hypnosis (e.g., Barber, 1978) and is one of the premises of cognitive behavior therapy (see Wilson, 1978a), as Chapter Three will examine.

3

The *assumption* that imagination plays a most important role in sexual behavior has been made from the very beginning of sex therapy (Fromme, 1950; Hastings, 1963). Masters and Johnson (1970) coined the term "spectatoring" to describe the mental process by which the person compares actual performance with a mental model of what performance should be. Kaplan (1979) outlined the "turn off" mechanism as a mental process composed of negativistic images and affirmations or self-talk leading to the lack of sexual interest and desire. Imagination in sexual behavior was taken for granted. But even as late as 1979, the exact role of imagination in sexual behavior, including sexual desire, and how to channel mental images for the benefit of the sexual sufferer had not been systematically studied.

Here is where hypnotherapy meets sex therapy. Kaplan (1979) proposed the concept of "regression in the service of pleasure," but did not follow it to its experiential conclusion of self-hypnosis. No mental regression "in the service of the ego" (Kris, 1952) or "in the service of pleasure" (Kaplan, 1979) can take place without relinquishing the rational, logical, sequential mode of thinking—the "secondary-process thinking" of psychoanalysis (Rapaport, 1967)—since true, experiential, felt regression is a reliving of past events or attitudes, of ways of experiencing the world and reality. "Regression in the service of . . ." is a mental representation of previous experiences or attitudes. The more this experience precludes secondary-process thinking, the more purely regressive it is. In hypnosis, then, this phenomenon of "primary-process thinking" is essential and, because it is, the hypnotherapist stresses imagery, not reason; experience, not logic; affect, not understanding—though reason, logic, and understanding are not completely disregarded in hypnosis (see Fromm, 1977).

Consequently, in this first part, I intend to look closely at hypnosis and into the theoretical aspects of the use of hypnosis in sex therapy. But in order to do this, we first must take a look at the historical foundations.

1

The new

hypnosis

Most people, including professionals, think they know what hypnosis is all about. However, not even the experts agree on the meaning of hypnosis. To begin with, the word itself is a misnomer, since all the evidence points to the fact that whatever is described by that noun neither is sleep nor has very much to do with sleep (see Bowers, 1976, Chapter 8). Yet *hypnos* is sleep in Greek and many hypnotists talk about "going to sleep" and "waking up" when doing hypnosis. Somnambulism means "deep" hypnosis for many.

The construct hypnosis, then, acts as a shortcut to refer to something that is quite complicated, since the word can mean a special *state* of mental functioning, the *method* used to obtain that mental state, and also the *process* or experience of oneself in that "alternate state of consciousness."

Several authors have written splendidly about hypnosis in general (e.g., Weitzenhoffer, 1957; Hilgard, 1965; Barber, 1976; Frankel, 1976). Here I shall restrict myself to some issues of importance for the sex therapist interested in hypnosis.

CONCEPTUAL PROBLEMS

If we start by agreeing that the word hypnosis is a construct of something complex and mostly subjective, we may look into this thorny issue with an open mind. The view that has dominated this area of in-

5

quiry for many years is that hypnosis is *a state of alternate conscious-ness* called *trance*, which can be enjoyed only by those who have a personality *trait* called *hypnotizability*, after going through a ritual des-ignated as *induction* with the help and guidance of a hypnotist. For lack of a better description, I shall refer to this view as "Traditional," and those who espouse it as constituting the "Traditional School."

There are slight differences among theoreticians, as Barber (1976, footnote, p. 6) has indicated, regarding the state of hypnosis under the conditions just mentioned. It must be emphasized that this con-ception of hypnosis is still an assumption, not yet scientifically proven. In fact, the evidence is rather lean, as Ascher's (1977) summary of Barber's research indicates.

To briefly outline this position, the state of hypnosis or trance has been assumed to exist because of the wonders of hypnosis manifested in the extraordinary behaviors that "hypnotized" people engage in. Because certain behaviors (dependent variables) follow the hypnotic induction (independent variable) of certain individuals, and because these unusual behaviors do not usually occur without the hypnotic in-duction in those individuals responsive to *induction,* it is assumed that the induction puts people with a special personality trait or talent in a special mental state. A trance state can be induced by this ritual in those who are hypnotizable. While the Traditional School stresses the sequence from independent to dependent variables, the opposite group emphasizes the mediational or intervening variables. I shall refer to the latter as "The New Hypnosis." The mediational variables are *the inner processes,* both conscious and below the level of aware-ness (or subconscious), which produce "hypnosis" or which allow the individual to experience hypnosis.

Among the conscious processes are positive attitudes, explained as TEAM under my experiential definition of hypnosis presented later in this chapter. The subconscious processes are less clear and fall under what Rossi (Erickson and Rossi, 1979) has described as depotentiat-ing habitual frameworks and belief systems, triggering the unconscious search and facilitating the unconscious processes.

There may be more agreement than meets the eye between the two positions just described. One must remember that the Traditionalists accepted as a truism that no hypnosis can take place with uncooperative subjects. However, they did not develop the main consequence of this axiom, which is that hypnosis happens when a person allows it to happen. Orne (1977), identified with the Traditional School, addressed himself to crucial issues:

> The basic questions that need to be resolved are the differences between those individuals who have the skill of entering hypnosis and those who do not; the circumstances that facilitate and/or respectively inhibit the tendency to respond to hypnotic suggestion in those individuals who have the ability to do so; and the consequences of being in hypnosis for an individual's psychological functioning (pp. 19-20).

Three points are worthy of note in the above statement: First, Orne refers to *the skill* of entering hypnosis, not to the trait of hypnotizability, much like The New Hypnotists. Second, he mentions the *circumstances* conducive to hypnosis, allowing us to focus on the most important "circumstance," namely, the hypnotist who can facilitate or inhibit the hypnotic experience. And third, Orne stresses the subjective aspect of the experience, which is also particularly considered by The New Hypnosis.

The evidence presented by Barber, Spanos and Chaves (1974) shows *the ability* to enter hypnosis to be a positive mental set, as described in the next section. Other authors (Diamond, 1974, 1977, a, b, 1978; Kinney and Sachs, 1974; Reilley et al., 1980; Sachs and Anderson, 1967) emphasize the skills and learned, cognitive behavior, grounded in the research done to modify hypnotic responsivity and that of cognitively oriented experimentalists, such as DeStefano (1977), Katz (1978, 1979; Katz and Crawford, 1978), and Spanos (1971; Spanos and Barber, 1972).

The Traditionalists, on the other hand, have relied on the hypnotizability *trait*, as ascertained by the classical scales of hypnotizability (Weitzenhoffer and Hilgard, 1959, 1962; Shor and Orne, 1962), about which more will be mentioned subsequently.

After considering the subjects, Orne looks at the circumstances of hypnosis. Besides the flexibility of the clinician—Erickson calls it "the utilization approach" (Erickson and Rossi, 1979)—The New Hypnosis considers the subject's willingness to "think with" and imagine the things that are suggested. This is, in essence, a willingness to learn, the concept so frequently mentioned by Erickson. That willingness, coupled with practice, produces the hypnotic effects. On the other hand, the Traditional School is vaguer on this score because the evidence shows that the induction ritual does not account for the hypnotic effects, as Bernheim (1964) demonstrated almost a century ago, since the same effects happen spontaneously, albeit rarely.

Regarding the subjective consequences of hypnosis, both "schools" are pretty much in agreement. Orne (1977) talks about the "transcendence of normal volitional capacities"; Hilgard (1965) mentions the seven characteristics of the hypnotic state, including changes in reality orientation, attention, and suggestibility. The New Hypnosis, nevertheless, focuses more on the cognitive effort, the permission one gives him/herself to experience different sensations or a different internal orientation, stressing the idiosyncratic meaning of the experience—one "let's himself go."

Among the subjective consequences of hypnosis, I like to include the functions of the parasympathetic division of the autonomic nervous system. This is not sufficiently emphasized by many authors, perhaps because hypnosis is not the only way of allowing the parasympathetic to function freely. Shames and Sterin (1978) are among the few who have stressed this aspect of hypnosis. They remind us that in hypnosis the stored-up tensions from the sympathetic response start to be released, allowing the parasympathetic to take over. Hypnosis could, then, be described as a mental process which *gives the parasympathetic a chance.* *

But, by definition, we cannot give the parasympathetic a chance by sheer effort and willpower. This only engages the sympathetic further. The change into parasympathetic functioning comes about by itself, only when one gives up the effort to change and *allows* the parasympathetic to take over. This constitutes the receptive state Wick

---

* I am by no means implying that *all* parasympathetic states are positive and pleasurable. Some of these parasympathetic states become negative and unpleasant, as in the case of apathy, emotional passivity and some forms of depression.

(1981) has studied. According to her, receptivity is the characteristic of the state of hypnosis. Receptivity is one of the three states of transactional direction, which are: inflow (receptivity), output (activity) and no-activity (passivity). It seems, therefore, that the assessment of autonomic nervous system functioning may provide an objective measure of these three states of transactional direction and, consequently, of hypnosis as a state of increased parasympathetic functioning.

From all the above, one can see the significance of Orne's definition, which can also be adopted by The New Hypnosis: Hypnosis is "that state or condition in which appropriate suggestions will elicit distortions of perception and memory" (pp. 18–19) (which Orne equates to hypnotic phenomena). Sarbin (1950) had defined hypnosis as a role that is played with such conviction as to become totally compelling to the individual. If we do not understand Sarbin's role assumption as being a conscious effort on the part of the subject, his definition coincides to a great extent with Orne's—the "believed-in imagining" of Sarbin and Coe (1972). The New Hypnosis will deny that "appropriate suggestions" elicit anything. The subject's willingness to experience him/herself differently is what produces change.

AN EXPERIENTIAL DEFINITION OF HYPNOSIS

There are conceptual issues, indeed, that divide the two current approaches to hypnosis among professionals. But regardless of these disagreements, it seems clear that we are justified in referring to hypnosis as *a state in which the critical mental faculties are temporarily suspended and the person uses mainly imagination or primary-process thinking.* The level of hypnosis, its *depth,* depends on how involved the person is in his/her imagining.

The analogy is closer to an intense type of daydreaming, rather than to sleep or to "being out of it." Thus, *when I let myself go into a goal-directed daydream to the extent that I dissociate myself from my surrounding reality and become engrossed in my inner reality, I am in an alternate state of awareness which is called hypnosis.* Because of this view, I consider many of the techniques used by the cognitive behavior therapists (see Chapter Three) as definitely hypnotic in nature.

As can be seen, there are four elements in my descriptive definition. First, "I let myself go" emphasizes the cognitive, volitional aspect, sometimes referred to as "giving myself permission," which presupposes the positive mental set mentioned earlier. Letting go means
trust in one's own inner mind capabilities and in the "hypnotist" one is
working with. In some cases, as when imagination is minimal (see the
section in this chapter on Imagination and Hypnosis), the main factor
operating in this internal dynamic of "letting oneself go" is the trust the
client has in the clinician using hypnosis—or, in the case of self-hypnosis, the trust in one's subconscious processes of mind.

Since clinical hypnosis, in most cases, involves a teamwork between therapist and client, the acronym TEAM may be helpful to indicate the *trust, expectations, attitudes,* and *motivation* necessary for
hetero-hypnosis. *Trust* refers to the client's perception of the clinician
as a decent and honest human being and as a competent professional.
The *expectations* must be realistic, as opposed to miraculous—looking forward to an interesting experience of learning about one's self
and of personal enrichment. This will elicit an *attitude* of cooperation,
not of challenge or defiance, which gives the client the *motivation* to
learn this new way of using one's mind and to benefit from it.

Second, a "goal-directed daydream" considers the reason why
one engages in this activity, or the goals one has for experiencing hypnosis. In the case of sex therapy, one may get so involved in erotic
imagery that it, in itself, triggers one's desire for sexual activity—a
method which has been very effective in cases of sexual abulia (Araoz,
1980, a). When one lapses spontaneously into an intense daydream,
this is also hypnotic, but without a goal or purpose chosen by the subject in a conscious way. The goal-directed daydream idea emphasizes
the self-control aspect of hypnosis (Katz, 1977), namely, the fact that
I decide to use hypnosis for a particular purpose, in order to attain a
specific goal.

Third, "dissociation from my surrounding reality" refers to the natural consequences of being occupied in the goal-directed daydream.
The more involved one is in it, the less concerned one becomes with
the things that are immediately around—those distracting stimuli
from the circumjacent environment. The dissociation, then, is in no
way a loss of control; rather, it is an enjoyable freedom to let the envi-

ronment go, so that one can concentrate on one's inner reality and experience.

This leads to the fourth, and last, element of my definition, but perhaps the most important. "To be engrossed in my inner reality" corresponds to the healthy madness or constructive craziness of hypnosis. Because I allow myself to be so engrossed in my inner reality, I experience all sorts of nonreality-oriented phenomena: I don't feel a pain that a few minutes earlier was "real"; I become a four-year-old and experience myself as the child I was many years ago; I see as possible and attractive something that for a long time created fear in me (think of any sexual activity); I smell flowers that are not there; I see myself then when I am overweight. . . . I can go constructively crazy.

Hypnosis, then, takes place when my critical faculties, my logic, my reality-oriented thinking are set aside, and I plunge into cartoon-like thinking or imagination where nothing is impossible.*

SUGGESTIBILITY AND HYPNOSIS

Is hypnosis the same as suggestion? This debated issue divides many authors who don't distinguish between the different types of suggestions, namely, *ordinary suggestions* ("please take a seat," "let me have your coat," "follow me this way"), *non-conscious suggestions* (yawning, a musical tune, many "tricks" of the advertisement industry such as liquor posters for commuters on the way home), and *hypnotic suggestions*.

Hypnotic suggestions are given to the person (or to oneself) when in hypnosis. They are received directly by the subconscious mind only if they are ego-syntonic and idiosyncratic. That is the reason why hypnotic suggestions are not any arbitrary ideas introduced to a person regardless of individual values, history, culture, religious convictions, and the like. Bernheim (1964) already warned us of this crucial point:

---

*This, incidentally, is one of the real dangers of hypnosis and one area where abuses may take place: a person may use hypnosis to escape external reality to the extent that s/he avoids obligations or responsibilities, or a person may get so involved in hypnosis that s/he stays in his/her inner world, denying the external one. Psychosis, from this point of view, is the extreme of negative self-hypnosis.

The suggestions given in hypnosis must fit the person and be uniquely tailored to that individual. Lack of success in hypnosis is often the result of a disregard for this basic principle. Erickson (Haley, 1967) was so dramatically successful because of his extreme sensitivity to the uniqueness of each person he worked with.

Hypnotic suggestions must activate inner resources that the person already has, at least germinally. As Bowers (1978) put it so well, they are the ideas the person listens to with "the third ear." Therefore, rather than to confuse suggestibility with hypnosis, one must realize that in hypnosis the person becomes more suggestible or is better at accepting suggestions that are idiosyncratic and ego-syntonic. The fascinating experiment conducted by Evans (1979), who administered suggestions to sleeping subjects, proved that those who were better at hypnosis were better at accepting the sleep-administered suggestions. Since the suggestions given had to do with the production of dreams and the content of the same, they were respectful of the subjects' individuality.

One of the great advantages of using hypnosis in clinical work lies in the fact that in a trance state one is free to accept positive, healthy, constructive suggestions without the interference of intellectualizations, objections, excuses, and rationalizations. That suggestibility correlates with hypnosis is accepted by all researchers and practitioners in hypnosis.

IMAGINATION AND HYPNOSIS

All experts agree on the fact that there is a high correlation between these abilities (Hilgard, 1970): Subjects good at imagining are also good at hypnosis. The New Hypnosis stresses the need to train those who find it difficult to imagine. Once they have become adept at imagining, they are ready for hypnosis. As all physically healthy humans with average intelligence can learn to speak and read, so too can they learn to use imagination and hypnosis.

Chapter Three will discuss at more length the meaning of imagination or mental images, pointing to the fact that I do not limit imagery to mental pictures. Any of the inner senses activated in order to access the necessary information to decode one's sensations—be it auditory, kinesthetic, gustatory, olfactory, or visual—is encompassed by *mental imagery* or imagination. *Imago* means reflection or representation in Latin.

Therefore, for a healthy, normal human being, imagination is part of his/her natural attributes, and hypnosis is a method by which imagination can be used most effectively. When imagination is used effectively, the person is in hypnosis, according to my experiential definition presented earlier. However, the use of imagination may be very subtle, since images, as was just explained, may not necessarily be "pictures."

Erickson was undoubtedly the master of indirection. In several of his cases (Erickson, 1966), he succeeded in using hypnosis without picture images, but activating, through indirection, other inner senses and experiences. In the case of the woman who was planning to become a professional harpist but had chronic sweating of her palms and fingers, Erickson (Erickson and Rossi, 1979) discovered the connection with a sexual dysfunction and dealt with both problems—hand sweating and sex—by a process of two-level communication, employing auditory imagery when he suggested that she listen in her mind to her favorite piece of music.

While she was consciously concentrating on the imaginary music, her inner mind was capturing Erickson's sexual associations, as the following quote indicates (my emphasis): "*You are in position* to start (pause) listening to some part (pause) of that (pause) *piece of music . . .* Just *listen slowly* to it (pause) and really, *thoroughly enjoy* that piece of music . . . Your unconscious mind will understand (pause) things that you can't understand" (Erickson and Rossi, 1979, pp. 150-151). Erickson's clinical hypothesis of a sexual problem masked by the symptom could have been wrong. Nothing would have been endangered in that case, however, since the client's subconscious would not have made the correction and would have missed the sexual implications. His indirection through the imaginary music the client was listening to in her mind became both a diagnostic and therapeutic tool for Erickson.

In most cases, imagination can be used to start the unconscious process, as Erickson did with this woman. Imagination can also be the main activity in hypnosis: By imagining oneself cured, the person can really activate immunological processes that will accelerate his/her cure (LeShan, 1977; K. R. Pelletier, 1979). The image of a healthy self triggers subconscious forces that *produce* a healthy self (A. M. Pelletier, 1979). The popular books on *mental* tennis or any other sport use basically this technique (Nideffer, 1976).

WHAT IS HYPNOSIS?

My initial definition—functional, rather than static; experiential, rather than conceptual—facilitates the understanding of what is meant by communication with the subconscious as being a characteristic of hypnosis. When a person lets him/herself go and becomes totally engrossed in his/her inner reality, s/he is suspending the critical and logical mental functions and is in touch with the wealth of memories, perceptions, experiences, wisdom, things learned, and resources which are usually untapped, "disconnected" from consciousness. While the individual is in touch with the subconscious, new psychological connections are made—like the harpist with the perspiring hands. The inner reality is not limited only to what one started to imagine initially in a conscious way. Once one has become engrossed in one's inner reality through the temporary dissociation from the external stimuli, the subconscious may take over—much as when we dream—and continue its activity in surprising directions.

Hypnosis, then, is also a method for getting in touch with one's subconscious mind. If sexual difficulties (as we shall see later in the book) are related to subconscious "thinking," hypnosis becomes a therapeutic intervention that cannot be neglected by a sex therapist. But I must underline that The New Hypnosis is not the traditional, ritualized, mysterious, and esoteric type about which most people, including professionals, feel apprehensive.

The New Hypnosis stresses self-mastery rather than "being asleep"; affective or visceral learning rather than obedience to suggestions given by the hypnotist; practice of a skill rather than isolated experience of a trance state produced during the clinical sessions with the hypnotist (see Diamond, 1978).

There is no question that in hypnosis the person is in a different mental state than when, let's say, paying bills or talking to a business associate about a problem. But there is a different mental state also when one is angry or sexually aroused or frightened or physically sick or very happy and excited about something. The alternate state of hypnosis, different from that of ordinary awareness, is controlled by parasympathetic functions, unlike in the "altered" state of unusual anger or happy excitement. The more we allow the parasympathetic to take over, the more we experience hypnosis. We are in a different state, both mentally and physiologically, than when we are actively engaged, under sympathetic control. This alternate awareness is the essence of hypnosis, which many call *trance*. As long as one understands that trance does not mean "being out of it," the word is as imperfect and as convenient as *hypnosis* itself.

The points of agreement between the two main trends in the current conceptualization of hypnosis are very important and basic. However, at the practical level, the difference is vast, considering the new stress on self-hypnosis and skill practice, just to mention one point.

Because the main locus of control for the Traditionalists is the hypnotist, they do not insist on self-hypnosis as often as the New Hypnotists do. In many cases, self-hypnosis was not taught until many sessions with the hypnotist had been spent. The New Hypnosis, on the other hand, considering the locus of control primarily in the subject, underlines the *need* for self-hypnosis, for tireless practice, from the very beginning. Most often I record in an audiotape what I say to the person in hypnosis so that s/he may practice faithfully at home until our next meeting. In fact, the whole experience is often presented as one of self-hypnosis—not hypnosis—with the admonition that without practice it is useless.

To summarize this section, I definitely have no objection to describing hypnosis as a state of mind different from many other mental states, including ordinary consciousness. I prefer to avoid the analogue of trance because of its possible misleading implications, especially in clinical work.

Regarding the nature of hypnosis, the evidence shows that it is a method of communicating with the subconscious mind and of triggering mental or physiological processes regulated subconsciously. It is a way of using subconscious activities for one's benefit. In this sense it is a different way of experiencing oneself, compared to the ordinary left-hemispheric, reality-oriented way. Thus, as was mentioned at the beginning of this chapter, hypnosis is (a) a method to get into (b) a different mental state which allows us (c) to experience ourselves as subconscious beings but with the ability to manipulate this inner personal wealth intentionally. Or, as Brown (1980) put it in terms of *units of consciousness*, in hypnosis "there is a dissociation of one complete unit-universe of consciousness, functionally isolated from nearly all other units of consciousness and their constituent elements of associated elements of perceptions, memories, judgment and logic associations" (p. 277). It is easy to perceive in her statement the echoes of Hilgard's (1977a, b) neodissociation explanation, which is intimately connected with the issue of suggestions in and out of hypnosis. Interpreting dissociation as a matter of degree, Hilgard (1977a) demonstrated that many dissociated activities take place outside of hypnosis; only when they are sufficiently widespread, do they imply "a change of the total state" or hypnosis.

One question that can be raised about this understanding of hypnosis is related to the hypnotizability scales. In experimental hypnosis, these scales provide the uniform measurement necessary to study hypnosis. The criterion of hypnotizability is the score obtained in the scales. But in clinical hypnosis, the real issue is not hypnotizability— since we know that all healthy, normally intelligent persons can use hypnosis—but rather *hypnotizing-ability*. The burden of proof is on the clinician, not on the client. Consequently, to use the same criterion in clinical hypnosis as in experimental hypnosis is to limit unnecessarily one's clinical possibilities. Even Weitzenhoffer (1980), who authored one of the well-known hypnotizability scales, has since raised questions about them.

People suffering from psychogenic sexual dysfunctions are not using cognitions properly. They are reinforcing their problem with their *thinking*. As Chapter Three will explain, *cognition* is used to comprise all reality-oriented mental activities involved in assessment, interpretation, and planning, namely, not just thoughts, beliefs, and ideas, but also imagery and feelings. These clients do need sex therapy, as it is commonly understood, but they also need desperately a new mental skill to clear their "thoughts," to manipulate their inner personal wealth, to use their subconscious mental processes for their own benefit. When the sex therapist adds hypnosis to his/her treatment, the effectiveness of the latter is increased and the length of therapy is shortened (Araoz, 1980b).

The use of hypnosis adds the missing dimension in traditional sex therapy, namely, the intervening variable of the client's "thinking." This book does not advocate the dismissal of the exercises prescribed to the person or couple suffering from sexual dysfunctions, following the teachings of Masters and Johnson. It does advocate *the addition of hypnosis*—as it is understood in this book—to those exercises and practice.

Before proceeding to study more technical aspects of hypnosis in the next few sessions of this chapter, it is important to remember that when I mention hypnosis, I always have in mind self-hypnosis. In other words, I never use hypnosis without teaching the client to practice it at home, with the audiotape made especially for him/her. Many experts have stated it again and again: Hypnosis is always self-hypnosis—a concept especially useful in sex therapy in order to help clients regain mastery and control over an area of their life that feels beyond their power.

HYPNOTIC INDUCTION

The New Hypnosis deemphasizes *the ritual* of induction. It prefers to refer to it as "setting events for skill utilization" (Diamond, 1978) or as "think-with instructions" (Barber, Spanos, and Chaves, 1974) or as "training inductions" (Katz, 1977).

Despite this deemphasis, induction cannot be dismissed lightly. It is the process by which a person moves from the ordinary way of using his/her mind to hypnosis. As such, it usually comprises two elements, at least for the uninitiated client. These elements are instructions on what hypnosis is all about, and some technique to move from the ordinary way of using one's mind (from ordinary thinking) to the other, where *one lets oneself go into a goal-directed daydream to the extent that one dissociates oneself from one's surrounding reality and becomes engrossed in one's inner reality*—our definition of hypnosis.

When the client requests "hypnosis," I explain that s/he is to engage in a goal-directed daydream, that this is a way of emphasizing experiential thinking as opposed to logical and critical thinking. This explanation helps to avoid the misconceptions the person may bring about hypnosis from stage hypnosis and movies depicting it. At this point I may suggest that the client imagine something very familiar to him/her, such as one's bedroom. If the person is not able to "visualize" his/her bedroom, I may ask whether the client is able to recall any smells connected with the bedroom, any sensations associated with the bedroom, any sounds that come to mind when thinking of the bedroom. This approach follows Bandler and Grinder's (1979) view of our inner representational systems, as will be explained in Chapter Three when discussing mental images. The moment the person responds positively to one of the inner senses—say, s/he is able to associate some smells with the bedroom—s/he is encouraged to make that inner olfactory representation even sharper and clearer. Then, using the principle of overlap, the person is invited to imagine the source of that smell and, if unable yet to visualize it, to touch it or feel it with his/her hands or any other part of the body. In this way, the person is given an opportunity to realize what is meant by experiential thinking, as opposed to logical, critical, rational thinking. In this way, also, the person is immediately instructed on enlarging his/her inner experiences by slowly moving from his/her preferred representational system—in the above case, smell—to other "channels" of the inner reality. To repeat, if the person is preferentially auditory (let's say), other inner senses are introduced—touch, smell, vision, taste—in order to make the goal-directed daydream of hypnosis more vivid and effective. Thus, new representational systems are made to overlap with the person's preferred one. (Incidentally, many of the Traditionalists have stressed the importance of involving as many inner senses as possible in the hypnotic experience and recommend techniques for vivid imagining (Weitzenhoffer, 1957).)

All of the above is part of the preparation for hypnosis or the instructions given the candidate to benefit from the experience of hypnosis. Once the person has successfully used imagination in the manner described above, the hypnosis practice is an extension of that "preparation." It can start by suggesting a relaxed and comfortable position, the closing of one's eyes and the listening to the hypnotherapist's voice. One may suggest attention to the person's breathing or start immediately by the inner representation of a pleasant and secure scene.

What about such things as concentration on one hand, so that the person may feel that hand to be very light and rising spontaneously? This traditional induction maneuver and others, like swinging a shiny pendulum in front of the person's eyes, can be helpful, especially if the person expects those actions to be part of hypnosis. But they are not necessary. As a matter of fact, I find them counterproductive in most cases, because by using these maneuvers, one is conveying the message that there is something mysterious about hypnosis and, also, that the hypnotist has some power over him/her. I want to emphasize the subject's or client's involvement, activity, and responsibility in hypnosis.

I don't find it useful to spend any time with explanations unless the client seems to have misconceptions about hypnosis. The sooner I can get to the experiential, non-critical mental activities, the more effective I find the process. So, my view of induction is very literal, namely, to "guide" the client "into" a different state of awareness than the critical, intellectual, rational awareness s/he is familiar with. This new state of awareness is effected *inductively,* namely from particular samples of the client's behavior to a general manner of thinking. The particular samples of the client's behavior are, e.g., unconscious choice of words and phrases which betray a preferential sensory channel—gestures, facial expressions, breathing rate, any slight movements. I may suggest that the person become aware of such "behavior" and use it in the way described in the section on Objections in this chapter and, again, at more length, in Chapter Six. Through these behaviors clients find their alternate reality. I don't impose it on them. I don't even contaminate their alternate awareness by imposing my own "induction technique" on them. On the contrary, I observe clients keenly and pace them carefully, meeting them where they are and proceeding from there to a richer inner experience.

Therefore, induction to me is not a formalized technique. I know that I am using an induction because I am utilizing a piece of the client's behavior to get to the unique mode of thinking of this unique human being, respecting his/her individual mental frame of reference. But I don't have to announce hypnosis and proceed with an "induction."

In practice, induction means the clinician's sensitivity to the client's existential world, so that the former may assess the latter's "availability for trance" (Erickson and Rossi, 1979). If we consider the research on the *ultradian cycle* (Hiatt and Kripke, 1975), it may be that humans are especially "available" for trance every 90 minutes or so. The clinician's task will be to detect the external signs of this rhythm, which up to recently was considered to take place only during sleep, as correlated with REM and dreaming.

Therefore, hypnotizability is a given rather than a question. The real question concerns the right moment for experiencing hypnosis. I speak about the concept of the ultradian cycle with clients who do not seem to succeed right away and encourage them to practice at home in order to find out when they are more available for trance. Having done this with more than 50 clients, for whom careful records have been kept, I am convinced of the existence of "special moments for hypnosis," as one client called them. Rather than finding the "right moment," one becomes aware of the signals of this brief rest period that recurs every 90 minutes or so. These are distractions of attention, tiredness, hunger, restlessness, awareness of changes in temperature, spontaneous daydreaming, and the like. Hiatt and Kripke have measured physiological changes taking place at those 90-minute intervals.

This fascinating discovery of the ultradian cycle should not lead us to believe that people are not available for trance at other times as well. What the ultradian pattern seems to mean is that at those times the organism welcomes the opportunity to enter an alternate state of awareness *more readily* than at other times.

HYPNOTIZABILITY OR HYPNOTIZING-ABILITY?

This is, perhaps, the most heated point of controversy between the two trends in the current thinking about hypnosis. All the Traditionalists insist on the need to establish or assess hypnotizability. "Is this a good hypnotic subject or not?" is an important question for them. The New Hypnotists, on the other hand, consider that any normally intelligent person with TEAM (see p. 10) can be trained to become a hypnotic candidate and can learn to use hypnosis. The evidence mentioned in the first section of this chapter confirms the initial hypothesis proposed by Diamond (1974) that responsiveness to hypnosis can be modified by several methods.

Rather than thinking of susceptibility to hypnosis or hypnotizability as a personality trait, we can consider it a skill, dormant in all healthy individuals, which can be developed by appropriate practice. This is a radical view for many Traditionalists, who claim that this position confuses a treatment strategy with hypnotizability, or suggestion ability with hypnosis. The fact remains, as Barber (1969) has demonstrated, that we are dealing with concepts, constructs, and abstractions to understand an experience which, in the final analysis, is essentially subjective.

The controversy about the modification of hypnotizability has been very alive in the last few years. But seldom do the authors remember to quote Weitzenhoffer (1957), who already a quarter of a century ago wrote:

> For a long time it has been believed that the more a subject is used in hypnotic experiments, the better subject he usually becomes. . . . Erickson finds that subjects who have experienced hypnosis many times over a long period of time, and who have also produced a great variety of hypnotic phenomena, are by far the better subjects. He sees this phenomenon as a learning process in which the subject learns to operate with increasing effectiveness in a hypnotic state. Subjects who lack such experience can be systematically taught various kinds of hypnotic behavior (p. 271).

This is a most interesting statement because it opens up the possibility of hypnotic training. Erickson's idea about increasing hypnotizability by means of practice is taken seriously enough by Weitzenhoffer to comment on it. But only many years later, mainly in the 1970s, has this issue been considered with the scientific rigor it deserves.

Since we are dealing with hypnosis in the practice of sex therapy, it seems that hypnotizability—in the sense of relatively stable personality trait—is a moot question. Clients should be encouraged to use their inner representational systems, and by this means they can get to that mental state where changes in values, beliefs, and perceptions are possible.

If one considers hypnosis as an alternate but *natural* state of awareness or consciousness, *any person with TEAM* (trust, expectations, attitudes, motivation) can be a good subject. It is the worker's task to pay close attention to the clients' clues in order to detect their representational systems. Making them good hypnotic subjects will consist in observing and pacing the clients closely so that, starting from their representational system, clients can be helped to activate other inner senses. Then their increased absorption in the inner reality diminishes and weakens their "connection" with external stimuli. Their awareness has changed—has been altered; they are in an alternate state of consciousness.

The current understanding, still rejected by the Traditionalists, is that any normal individual of average intelligence *can be taught* to experience hypnosis. Perhaps the issue of hypnotizability should be altered in order to question the clinician's ability to use hypnosis properly. We should talk about *hypnotizing-ability,* which is what perhaps Freud lacked (see Gravitz and Gerton, 1981), and because of which his followers, as a group, felt discomfort with hypnosis.

DEPTH OF HYPNOSIS

There is danger of confusion when the analogue is taken for the real thing to which it refers. In hypnosis, some take the trait of hypnotizability, or the depth of hypnosis, as if it were a real thing, rather than an inadequate attempt at describing a unique and subjective experience. Perhaps we should change the whole language of hypnosis and talk, for instance, about hypnotic *height,* rather than depth, or *superconscious,* instead of subconscious. In fact, with some patients I have purposely used expressions like "superconscious," "getting higher into hypnosis," and such, with the same success that the traditional words have produced.

In spite of many arguments from the conservative wing in hypnosis, Tart (1979) makes a good case for preferring self-reports of depth to any other more objective assessments. In clinical practice, the more a person lets him/herself go into a goal-directed daydream and so on, as we saw before, the deeper s/he is into the experience of hypnosis. In sex therapy, especially, the most important therapeutic element is the client's change in cognitions obtained by means of the newly learned skill of hypnosis. Even in so-called light states of hypnosis, clients obtain therapeutic benefits from using their minds constructively, positively, filling their thoughts with self-enhancing imagery and giving themselves beneficial suggestions.

The confusion between experimental and clinical hypnosis appears again in the issue of depth, as in the issue of hypnotizability. Both concepts are useful and even necessary in *studying* hypnosis, but not in the *application* of hypnosis for therapeutic purposes.

A CASE ILLUSTRATION

The professional should learn as much as possible about hypnosis, but, in applying it to the client, s/he should use it naturally, as part of one's communication, without complicated explanations, which often confuse and scare the client. An illustration might be in order.

Del is a 30-year-old man, married for three years and having a good loving relationship with his wife, who complains about erectile dysfunction—he has a strong erection at the beginning of lovemaking but loses it a few minutes later and cannot become erect after that. After ascertaining that this is not a medical problem, and because my preferential mode of therapeutic communication is hypnosis, I have several choices. I will, at this point, illustrate one of these choices.

The information given so far is enough to proceed "hypnotically." I would simply ask him, as a first step, to experience himself in his inner mind having that sexual difficulty—to really get into the misery and any other feelings that he usually experiences. I want to be sure that he is reliving his problem. When his face, general body tension, his breathing, and his own report tell me that he is experiencing fully his sexual difficulty, I interrupt (step two) and ask him to think of a situation—not necessarily sexual—which is the complete opposite of the former one, a situation in which he has the ability to enjoy himself, to be sure of himself, to act optimally. I would also encourage him at this point to increase all the good, positive feelings generated by that situation. Then (step three) I would ask him to transfer all these good feel-

NLP

NLP

ings to the sexual situation. This transfer I would repeat as many times as needed to effect the new mental picture of sex with enjoyment and without worry. In other words, the positive feelings can "correct" the mental picture of his sexual "failure" and make his "mental sex" enjoyable and fun.

This schematic illustration is enough to underline the point I am trying to make: *that to use hypnosis you don't have to announce hypnosis.* If hypnosis is the mental state in which one has suspended the function of his/her critical faculties and is engaged in experiential thinking, the above description is all hypnosis. Del changes his state of consciousness by getting into this exercise. Through my help he discovers a new mental resource he was not using before. In so doing, he is programming himself to succeed, to enjoy, to act naturally and without worry. The more he and I can focus on the new "program," the weaker the old program becomes. Once he has learned this technique with me, he is encouraged to practice it alone many times and to really immerse himself in the good feelings of the positive mental picture. The result, as recent data indicate, is an overwhelming success (see Barber, 1980).

The use of hypnosis without announcing hypnosis was one of the remarkable features of Erickson's uniqueness in his last years. This is justified because all deeply human communication is hypnosis. For example, when you tell me in dramatic detail what happened to you in your last trip to Europe, you are intent *on changing my awareness.* You are trying to place me in an alternate state of cognition so I can experience in my mind what you experienced in your trip. *You are inducing a new state of consciousness in me.* If you succeed, my surrounding reality weakens temporarily while I am partaking of your reality. Your reality becomes temporarily paramount for me.

The ancient hypnotic art of storytelling has been considered for centuries effective in transporting an audience to a different reality. The story allows the listeners "to leave behind" the weariness of a humdrum existence. The story becomes "real" and the surrounding reality remote and unimportant—at least for a while.

In a more active way, a thorough sexual involvement is hypnotic inasmuch as one is absorbed by the experience, as Mosher (1980) pointed out. While the sexual "reality" lasts, the ordinary orientation to mundane concerns is weakened.

In other words, my mental absorption becomes my reality. What I
think is what I am—Cogito, ergo sum. Or, as Bach (1977) put it, "We
magnetize into our lives what we hold in our thoughts." Hypnosis at
its best! We change outwardly through our cognitions.

HYPNOSIS: CLINICAL AND EXPERIMENTAL

All of the above emphasizes the need of the expert clinician to act
naturally, non-ritualistically. Regardless of the parameters used by the
researcher to establish the presence of hypnosis, the clinician can use
the basic mechanisms of hypnosis in order to help people change.
The researcher must measure results with mathematical exactitude;
the clinician measures them by individual outcomes. In research the
hypnotic effects are the dependent variables; for the clinician, what
happens *after* hypnosis, namely, the results in the person's life, are
the only valid dependent variables. So, in the case of Del, the fact that
he changed after hypnosis and was able to enjoy what before had
become a source of anxiety is the most important proof that there was
hypnosis and that it worked. The empirical proof requested by the clinician is different than that of the researcher. Confusion has arisen recently when, due to the demands of consumerism and the greater
awareness of accountability, clinicians tried to become researchers
and to do both simultaneously.

The final proof of any therapy is its long-term outcome. Many clinicians, like myself, who had not used hypnosis initially, have found
that clients change more quickly and more radically with this new
tool, and the changes are more lasting. Regardless of the theoretical
issues, when a clinician sees that hypnosis works, s/he considers it a
valuable intervention. For most clinicians—and many of us are "con-
verts" from other approaches or theoretical schools—the comparison
between one's ante-hypnosis and post-hypnosis therapeutic work is a
strong enough argument in its favor. More clients have been helped
more rapidly and with more lasting effects with hypnosis than before I
used hypnosis. Furthermore, the clinical work has become more exciting, more creative, more varied. So hypnosis benefits not only the
clients but the clinician as well.

These grand claims in favor of clinical hypnosis must be proven.
But as Lieberman (1977) points out in a paper that should be read

and reread by all serious hypnotists, it is difficult to validate claims if the method we use to find the evidence is inadequate. Lieberman complains about the experimental method itself—a heretical act for many which, in itself, would place the author among the outcasts. Among other very important points, Lieberman mentions the "question of whether we have any right to generalize conclusions from laboratory experiments with a recorded standard induction on college students to all hypnotic inductions in all situations" (p. 64). This alone makes one wonder about research methodology in the social sciences in general and in hypnosis in particular, especially at a time when the current literature shows a growing awareness of the fact that large-group research paradigms—mimicking the physical sciences methods—seldom apply in clinical research. For instance, the $N = 1$ research model is recovering its scientific respectability after decades of marginal recognition because it can answer the real-life research questions asked by our direct work with individuals—clients, not Ss.

Although both types of research are "scientific," namely, concerned with validation, objectification, and utilization of data, the focus of clinical research is (should be?) on the growth and development of *the individual,* while the focus of experimental research is on *the mean* performance of a given population sample. The latter paradigm fails to consider individual behavior as lawful and systematic, and treats it as a variance of a random event. For instance, while the mean performance of a sample may improve with hypnosis, some individuals within that sample may deteriorate. Typically, the experimenter is interested in the sample, but the clinician is interested in the individuals who do not fall within one or two standard deviations from the mean. It may also happen that a handful of subjects in a group exposed to hypnosis for, say, sexual dysfunctions, show drastic improvement, thus producing a statistically significant change for the whole experimental group, which biases the results and, consequently, distorts the true effect of the procedure.

The results reported for the group would tell us nothing about a particular individual, thus becoming rather useless to the clinician. Indeed, this information may even become damaging if the clinician treats the individual who does not respond according to the "research" results as *deviant* or *abnormal.*

To stick doggedly to the traditional experimental design is to ignore current paradigms of research in the social sciences, such as intensive designs, SSR (same subject research), MBM (multiple baseline methods), empirical case studies, interrupted time series, and several others.

In line with the above, what I am reporting about hypnosis is based on my clinical experience. Each case, undoubtedly, must be treated idiosyncratically, but there are general rules of communication which must be used in order to make communication take place—as we cannot violate with impunity physical rules and then wonder about the "bad results." The "rules" we are referring to have to do with the way our mind works, as we indicated in the previous sections.

To me, one of the most important "rules" to keep in mind is that not all people "think" in the same way. The clinician must be aware of a client's preferential representational system.

NLP presup

EFFECTIVENESS OF HYPNOSIS IN SEX THERAPY

If faulty cognitions are a mediational variable in all psychogenic sexual dysfunctions, the method by which this can be altered must be welcomed as therapeutic. However, the evidence to prove the effectiveness of hypnosis in sex therapy is hard to gather because most reports are case studies without the control of subject variables (age, previous therapy, religion, etc.), without valid and reliable measurement procedures, and usually without a careful description of the structured therapeutic program used. Brown and Chaves (1980) reviewed 26 anecdotal reports. Unfortunately, they looked for the type of evidence one can find in experimental studies. One of their complaints, for instance, is that none of the reports studied isolated hypnosis as an independent variable, uncontaminated by other possible independent variables. Can this be done in clinical work? My comments in the previous section are relevant here also. As Brown and Chaves conclude, hypnotherapy—as opposed to experimental hypnosis—is not an easy area for research, if by research we restrict ourselves to the strict "scientific" method of finding out what is.

The impressive list of clinicians who have reported on the successful use of hypnosis in sexual dysfunctions can encourage the concerned practitioner to employ this method in his/her practice, especially in cases which have not responded successfully to other modalities of treatment.

The measurement of results in psychotherapy is a necessity, independent of current pressures from government and consumer agencies. We must know what effects our methods of intervention produce in given circumstances. But there seems to be growing confusion about the tools used for measuring the outcome of psychotherapy. For instance, the clamor for control groups may be an impossibility in clinical practice, at least with the exactitude obtained in the laboratory. The isolation of hypnosis as an independent variable may be another impossibility in clinical practice.

My argument in favor of hypnosis in sex therapy is based on several important facts, some of which have been mentioned earlier. First, cognitive control is achieved; second, relaxation from anxiety and stress is accomplished; third, consciousness of one's own "thoughts" for improvement or deterioration is raised; fourth, positive imagery is used for one's benefit; fifth, natural physiological processes are freed to function normally; sixth, the person acquires a new mental skill of self-control over his/her thoughts, the view of one's past, and physical functioning.

That these benefits generalize to other areas of functioning is known by all clinicians who use hypnosis. Often a person reports that s/he has practiced the new skill in the dentist's chair or in a situation that before was anxiety-producing and of which the clinician was not aware.

How long do these benefits last? Again, the consensus of those who are familiar with clinical hypnosis is that clients who are taught hypnosis use this skill—at least sporadically—many months and years after their clinical experience.

These facts cannot be denied on the basis that there is no scientific validation for them. Reality-testing is also a way of getting at the truth. And the reality of so many clinicians who practice hypnosis cannot be dismissed lightly.

One of the frustrations of traditional sex therapy has been the partners who do not practice the exercises prescribed or who do them half-heartedly. Hypnosis in sex therapy adds a new dimension which harmonizes the behavioral rehearsal with a new mental attitude.

The above comments do not imply in any way that we should give up attempts at validating and objectifying data pertaining to the effectiveness of hypnosis in sex therapy. On the contrary, every clinician could contribute to this goal by keeping careful records of what s/he has done with a particular client. And, once more, the difference between the experimenter and the clinician is that the latter cannot remain inflexibly faithful to his/her initial plan and, in sensitive response to the client's needs, must introduce new independent or mediational variables in the midst of treatment. This, obviously, is anathema in the laboratory but in the consulting office is a most frequent procedure. Not to do so would be to ignore the first rule of clinical work, namely, to help the client effectively.

OBJECTIONS

Many of the Traditionalists find an approach like mine confusing because it is less exact regarding issues of importance to them. The levels of depth are measured less carefully—mostly through self-reports; hypnotizability, scores to determine hypnosis, trance state vs. non-trance state, and other such issues are less carefully treated.

Perhaps the difference originates in the history of hypnosis itself. The Traditionalist school was in the mainstream of psychiatry with its unremitting emphasis on psychopathology, mental illness, and disease. First, Charcot (Freud's teacher and one of the great figures in psychiatry) and Janet, both of the Salpêtrière school of hypnosis, explained the phenomenon in terms of psychopathology—Janet talking of dissociation as an hysterical symptom. Beginning in the middle of the 19th century this was the strongest current in hypnosis. At the same time, in the French city of Nancy, Bernheim and Liébeault were developing an understanding of hypnosis which was nonpathological. They stressed suggestibility as the mental power to transform an idea into an act and hypnosis as a special state which heightens the susceptibility to suggestions. The Nancy school stressed health and normal mental functioning; the school of the Salpêtrière emphasized pathology. Later developments placed hypnosis in the Salpêtrière tradition. Only recently has the pendulum swung to the other side, with hypnosis being considered in terms of self-improvement, personal enrichment, and enhancement of the healthy aspects of being human, rather than as focusing on pathology in order to cure it.

From this book's point of view—a clinical orientation—many things in this field are the contribution of the Traditionalist school of hypnosis which follows Charcot and Janet, but most of the clinical uses of hypnosis fall more in line with the Nancy tradition of Bernheim and Liébeault.

SUMMARY

Although I have been writing about "schools of hypnosis," this is only a pragmatic designation. There is mutual respect between the two groups. As a matter of fact, the two professional societies of hypnosis in the U.S. publish contributions from both currents of thought and engage in healthy arguments about issues of disagreement.

At the risk of being repetitious, it should be stressed that the learning of hypnosis is essential in order to be able to do effective hypnotherapy. In this learning, induction techniques must be mastered, as well as deepening techniques, methods of giving hypnotic suggestions, and so on. But all that is like the rules on a paper—after you learn to write, you don't need them; or like the training wheels for a child learning to ride a bicycle—he is eager to discard them as soon as he has mastered the skill. My approach to hypnosis is naturalistic (Erickson and Rossi, 1979), avoiding as much artificiality as possible and starting always from the clients' reality and the mental system they are using to represent that reality.

Sensory and somatic awareness is for me the most natural way of helping a person change his/her awareness. I may start simply by asking the client to become conscious of any bodily sensations right here and now. Next, to see whether some "part" in him/her can increase these sensations. Then, to let those sensations act like a bridge and take him/her to anything in the past related somehow to the "problem" at hand. If something comes up—and most often this bodily awareness leads to meaningful material—we work on that, as I will explain in later chapters. If nothing happens, I suggest some somatic alteration, such as raising one or both arms, or changing the sitting position, or tensing up the whole body or part of it, before introducing the "bridge" concept.

In summary, one way of using hypnosis without announcing it to the client is by the three steps mentioned in the last paragraph:

First: Become aware of any sensations (or change bodily sensations artificially in order to become aware of any sensations).
Second: Intensify that awareness, those sensations.
Third: Let those sensations act as a bridge to take you to "something" related to your problem." *

In this manner, every normal person is hypnotizable, and the degree of hypnotizability becomes irrelevant. I work with the person's current subconscious processes and, consequently, it is unimportant to measure the depth of hypnosis. I see myself as a teacher who is showing the client new ways of using his/her mind, new ways of manipulating subconscious processes for his/her benefit.

The presence of TEAM (trust, expectations, attitudes, and motivation) is to me more important than clear and detailed intellectual understanding, on my part, of the person's problem. Once I ascertain that there is TEAM, I can proceed and all the necessary factual information will come up very promptly or—what may sound heretical to many psychotherapists—won't be needed at all. This process-focused approach to sex therapy will be explicated later. As I explained earlier, I also insist on the need to practice these "exercises" learned in the office and often give clients a tape recording made just for them so they can practice with it until they see me again.

Finally, my therapy is as structured as it can be so that it moves smoothly and cleanly. Many therapists dislike structured therapy:

---

*In the case of pain, one must obviously alter this procedure. I look for any slight expression of relief or statement of good sensations in the recent past. Then I ask the person to concentrate on that positive feeling, to increase it by experiencing him/herself in a pleasant, beautiful, healthy place. Once feelings of well-being are obtained, I continue to the "bridge" technique. Lutzker (1981), who uses hypnosis in a busy burn unit in a county hospital, agrees with the approach that looks for positive sensations.

They object that it may do away with spontaneity, it is artificial, and it is dehumanizing. All these objections are naive romantizations of therapy. The best musician is highly structured and, thanks to that structure, s/he can be creative, spontaneous, and unique. Language is most structured: We cannot arbitrarily use words in any "creative" order we want, disregarding syntax, if we desire to convey some meaning through those words. So, too, with hypnotherapy: The more structured it is, the more effective; the clearer the therapist is *in his/her own mind* as to the steps to follow, the quicker and more lasting the results.

But it is essential that the hypnotherapist see him/herself first and foremost as a clinician, not a researcher or experimenter. His/her main concern should be *the application and use* of hypnosis for clinical purposes, not *the study* of hypnosis. To confuse these two goals and interests when doing hypnotherapy produces bad research and worse therapy to the detriment of the clients. The two hats should be worn at different times and in different settings.

The next chapters will delve into the historical developments of hypnosis in sex therapy and consider the theoretical roots which validate this approach, adducing the evidence for using both hypnosis and sex therapy in the treatment of sexual dysfunctions.

2

Historical background

When looking at the development of hypnosis and sex therapy, a double approach is needed, namely, from the field of sex therapy and from that of hypnosis. In this chapter, I intend to review three main hypnotic approaches used even before sex therapy was accepted as a specialty and several other hypnotic techniques employed for sexual problems. Then, I will turn to sex therapy as such and look into its use of hypnotic techniques, from its beginning in the mid 1960s to the present.

The three authors to be studied first, Erickson, van Pelt and Beigel, are chosen because of two reasons. First, they described in detail their *modus operandi* as hypno-clinicians and they became well-known through their publications and professional contributions for using hypnosis for sexual dysfunctions. A third reason could be added, that the three started their contributions to the field in the 1930s.

These authors represent three different modalities of using hypnosis for sexual problems: Erickson triggers subconscious changes by indirect imagination techniques; van Pelt uncovers traumatic events of the past responsible for current difficulties; Beigel explores subconscious wishes and repressed needs, adding *in vivo* rehearsal when necessary.

INDIRECT IMAGINATION METHOD (ERICKSON)

The first detailed account of sex therapy through hypnosis was published by Erickson in 1935. His indirect imagination technique was applied to a man with premature ejaculation by creating a phobia related to the patient's problem. His subconscious connected the solution to the experimental phobia with his real problem and its solution. Erickson used the imagery of an ashtray and a cigarette, of the latter's heat and its damaging effect on the delicate glass ashtray, of a young woman alone with the patient offering him the ashtray she had artistically painted, to artificially create the phobia which was subsequently resolved. Through this indirect approach, Erickson helped the patient's subconscious do away with the anxiety associated with sexual intercourse manifested in premature ejaculation.

The emphasis on imagination in this case is obvious, though Erickson was not interested in stressing this aspect of hypnosis. Rather, he was investigating "the practicability of the use of hypnosis as a possible fertile technique for the laboratory study of the dynamics of human behavior" (Erickson, 1935, p. 48). Nevertheless, in using imagery rather than direct suggestions, the author was triggering primary-process thinking, dream-like material, through imagery. The unique feature of this case is that Erickson recognized the need to "readjust the personality" to overcome the psychogenic premature ejaculation, not by analyzing the patient's developmental dynamics, but, rather, by focusing his attention and mental imagery on a different "neurosis," that of being phobic of ashtrays. As Erickson put it:

> The heterosexual drives involved and the emotional forces at play in [the fabricated story used to create the artificial neurosis] — the man's attraction to the girl (sic), his desire to give her something and thereby to gain satisfaction for himself, the girl's display of herself by means of her artwork and the parallelism of the catastrophe of this contact with those of past heterosexual contacts — establishes a fair possibility of such identifications [namely, those feelings attached to the fabricated story and to his heterosexual difficulties] (1935, p. 36).

Erickson assures us that the young man in question overcame his sexual difficulty without any symptom substitution, even one year after the hypnotic experience. The author concedes that "the origin of the neurosis and its purposes and functions for the personality [were] not known" (p. 47), but the results indicated "definite and significant changes in his personality reactions" (p. 47), an argument hard to dismiss.

As I mentioned before, the concept of sex therapy was not yet developed in the early 1930s. Erickson treated this case as a symptom of some personality problem. However, he directed his clinical attention to the symptom, not to the analysis of the patient's personality. I believe that is the reason why he wrote about this case in research terms, calling it an experimental neurosis. One may speculate that Erickson's plan was to see whether this approach was effective and that he would have been prepared to employ a different technique had this one failed. As he put it:

> The technique of experimentation was suggested by the well-established clinical fact, both in medicine and in psychoanalytical therapy, that recovery from one illness (or conflict) frequently results in the establishment of a new physiological equilibrium (or "redistribution of libido") thereby permitting the favorable resolution of a second concurrent and perhaps totally unrelated illness (or conflict) (1935, p. 34).

He went on to state that "an intercurrent disease may exercise a favorable effect upon the original illness, for example, malaria in paresis" (p. 34). Based on these theoretical considerations he devised a "neurosis" symbolizing the original one and arousing similar emotions. This similarity of affect, he further assumed, would connect dynamically the two neuroses through a subconscious process of identification or of "absorption" of one problem upon the other. The resolution of the induced conflict was expected to transfer or generalize the abreactive process to the initial difficulty. Another possibility was that the resolution of the fabricated neurosis might reorganize the personality in such a way that the presenting symptom would no longer be necessary.

Many reports of successful hypnotherapy for sexual dysfunctions have been published since 1935, but very few of them give us any detailed account of what actually happened in the process of therapy. Erickson showed us what he did, how he did it, and why.

UNCOVERING AND SUGGESTION METHOD (VAN PELT)

Van Pelt (1949, 1958), on the other hand, took a more traditional approach, namely, that of exploring the origin or cause of the conflict. After discovering it, he used "new ideas" to "convince" the patient that the current reaction causing anxiety and producing symptoms was ineffective and dysfunctional. In his words:

> Concentration, or rather superconcentration, of the mind is hypnosis. Any idea implanted in the mind at this time, unless it is definitely against the subject's fundamental moral code, will probably be accepted. Once accepted it acts with the force of a hypnotic suggestion . . . (1958, p. 118).

Using this principle, van Pelt moved very swiftly once he had uncovered the cause for the current problem which, by the way, he did not believe was always found in early childhood but might be quite recent though repressed. His interventions consisted of direct suggestions to disconnect the past traumatic events from the current situation. In a curious case (van Pelt, 1958) of female sexual abulia, the wife was upset because of her husband's interest in "magazines for men" carrying pictures of beautiful women. Van Pelt found that as a child of five or six the patient had heard from her grandmother, who had a big varicose ulcer on her leg, that this injury was "your grandfather's fault. He makes me work too hard. All men are the same" (p. 193). This led the patient, at that early age, to say to herself: "'I must be careful of men —they might hurt me.' Following this she got the idea that if she felt 'numb and dead' then nobody could hurt her. . . . She had literally hypnotized herself into feeling 'numb and dead.' Small wonder it was that she had no real (sexual) feelings for her husband" (p. 193). Van Pelt's treatment consisted of "several sessions . . . directed to building up her morale and suggesting that she now was no longer a little girl and she would act and feel like a grown-up woman" (p, 194). Unfortunately, the author does not report in greater detail here how he used hypnosis to help this woman act and feel like a grown-up, sexually mature person. However, from his comments elsewhere (van Pelt, 1949) it is fair to speculate that he employed mostly mental imagery rather than simple commands or suggestions. The imagery used by van Pelt seems to have been of a mental rehearsal nature, not of the kind used by Erickson, as described earlier. This is how he described his clinical approach:

> The patient is instructed, while under only light hypnosis, to "form a picture" in his mind. He is asked to imagine a "3-D" cinema screen and to see himself "just like an actor" on this screen, playing a part. He is told that the picture looks "very real"—"3-D" in fact—and that he can see himself acting and looking the way he wants to look and act. Various scenes are suggested such as it is known that the patient will have to face in real life. In each, he is instructed to see himself "as in real life" always succeeding. . . . The patient is also instructed how to form these "success pictures" for himself, and it is stressed that he will only be able to see himself as he wants to be—"successful." Since the pictures give rise to the appropriate feelings it is not long before the patient begins to show the benefit of his private 3-D film shows (van Pelt, 1958, p. 51).

Van Pelt's approach is far from original nowadays but in the 1940s and 1950s this was innovative, especially coming from a recognized authority who became President of the British Society of Medical Hypnotists and Editor of the *British Journal of Medical Hypnotism*.

During this period Wolberg (1945) also wrote his by now classic work on hypnosis, describing the technique of visual imagery as an effective clinical tool for uncovering subconscious material. Psychoanalysts Brenman and Gill (1947) dared to bring hypnosis back to the couch, establishing solid theoretical reasons for their innovation. But van Pelt was one of the first authors to systematically describe how he used imagery for mental rehearsal and to familiarize the patient with the behaviors and feelings of the improved or cured state.

EXPLORATION AND *IN VIVO* REHEARSAL (BEIGEL)

Beigel (1972) offers a good example of very direct methods combined with careful psychodynamic concerns. His report is also one of the few early detailed explanations of what actually happened in the consulting room. Dealing with preorgasmic women, Beigel established a three-step approach to "inhibit the inhibitions" about sex, to "sensitize the psychogenically insensitive organs" and, in the process, to alter mental attitudes towards sexuality. Beigel started with the "hypnotic check-up," which served to correct misinformation given by the patient consciously. The author stated that often women would deny masturbatory practices out of shame or embarrassment at the conscious level but would admit them in hypnosis. "Just as dreams, daydreams and detailed memories serve as guides to the anesthesizing block and to the discovery of useable associations, so do they indicate the methods by means of which the obstacle to a healthy response is most likely to be overcome" (Beigel, 1972, p. 7).

Unlike other early hypnoclinicians, Beigel insisted on seeing the woman's sexual partner, engaging him as an *ad hoc* co-therapist. Beigel's method, during the second phase of treatment, consisted of training the partner in performing "the manual, oral and verbal functions" which are ego-syntonic to the woman.

> When [the man] has proved his skill on a dummy, the female is relaxed under hypnosis and a scene and location is suggested to which she is particularly receptive. . . . Actual sensitization starts with the stroking of the hands, the cheeks, the arms, the hair. The action is accompanied by flattering remarks and tender phrases on the part of the mate and by words descriptive of pleasant feelings on the part of the therapist who by that time has established a repertory of response patterns in the subject. She is encouraged to express the pleasantness of feelings in learned, or preferably, her own terms or gestures. In the beginning, the therapist directs feelings and responses of the female in trance; the later and more advanced stages are practiced in the privacy of the couple's home (p. 10).

A similar but very controversial approach, without the sexual partner's presence, is advocated by Macvough (1979), and not favored by reviewers such as Lerman (1980). A less polemic method was experimentally tested by Cox and myself (Cox and Araoz, 1977), as I shall explain later on, proving that imagery alone can produce orgasm. What was controversial about Beigel's technique was the foreplay activity in his presence. "As . . . stimulation proceeds from shoulder to breasts, hips, thighs and vulva, symptoms of excitement and feelings previously tested and evoked are intensified" (p. 10). He encouraged the "sighs, grunts and moans" as "the female is encouraged to let go, to blabber, to move her pelvis." Beigel believed that this latter aspect of the experience was important "in overcoming inhibitions [representing] at the same time a form of autosuggestion which stirs up emotions and helps generate or magnify the expected sensations" (p. 10).

Thus, Beigel's three stages consisted of initial interviews, practice sessions in the office and practice sessions at home, both conducted with the woman's sexual partner, as indicated. Throughout his report he stressed the need to search hypnotically for the subconscious reasons delaying the desired outcome, namely, the experience of orgasm. His rule was stated quite simply: "If [the desired effect] is not forthcoming within a reasonable time [sic], the reason for the delay may again have to be searched for, partly in the conscious state, partly in the state of hypnotic trance" (p. 11). What is a reasonable time was not explained and seems to be left to the judgment of the clinician. His method is another type of mental rehearsal (Beigel, 1963), rather than of hypnoanalysis.

OTHER HYPNOTIC METHODS

Though I have selected three authors because their clinical accounts are sufficiently detailed, there is a remarkable consistency in all the more global reports of those years: The success seems to be in direct proportion to the use of imagery, as opposed to direct suggestions. Some writers, like Crasilneck and Hall (1975), reflecting a rather psychoanalytical orientation, caution us of the possible unconscious meanings of sexual symptoms—advice which is hopefully unnecessary for the well trained therapist. These authors, however, assert unequivocally that "treatment by hypnosis of impotence and frigidity should always involve concurrent psychoanalysis or hypnoanalysis" (p. 279). If this means that the hypnotherapist should be ready to deal with underlying dynamics affecting the sexual dysfunction, I agree with their recommendation, which goes along with Kaplan's (1979) multicausal levels concept. This means, in her words, that "it is a basic

strategy of sex therapy to attempt to modify the immediate antecedents of the sexual symptom and to deal with more remote underlying
anxieties only if resistances arise in the course of treatment" (p. 145).
Other authors, however (see Kroger and Fezler, 1976), do not overem-
phasize the need for being aware of possible underlying psychodynamics, stating that "many forms of impotence have been treated by suggestion and directive hypnotherapy" (p. 140). But even they remind
us that "it is imperative to treat the interpersonal relationship between
husband and wife, not only the symptom-complex" (p. 165).

We observe, therefore, a double trend in the use of hypnosis for
sexual dysfunctions, namely, the direct approach—which seems to
be less favored by most authors—and the hypnodynamic one, considering the possible personality ramifications of the symptom as
such.

None of the three authors reviewed thus far advocates direct suggestion or commands for the removal of the sexual dysfunction. It is
interesting to note that both van Pelt and Beigel recommend that the
patient practice the hypnotic techniques at home, implying that practice would improve performance—the basic rule for developing skills
at a time when hypnosis was considered a trait and when great importance was given to the scales measuring a person's hypnotizability. As
we saw in Chapter One, there is mounting research and data stressing
the concept of hypnosis as a skill using a learning model, away from
the trait idea of old.

But, as mentioned when referring to Kroger and Fezler (1976),
direct suggestion *has* been employed for the treatment of sexual dysfunctions. None of the papers published explains in detail how these
direct suggestions are used and it seems that they are very seldom, if
ever, used without mental imagery. So, the question is whether suggestion alone is effective without imagery production to improve sexual dysfunctions.

In the papers considered below one finds this combination of suggestions with imagery as an hypnotic method of dealing with sexual
problems. I should remind the reader that because of the anecdotal
nature of most reports, it is not worthwhile to conduct a thorough
review of the literature. The few works mentioned are just a sample of
what has been published in this area.

Gilbert (1954) used hypnosis in treating homosexuality, which in those days was considered a pathological deviation. He suggested different hypnotic techniques when dealing with either passive or aggressive homosexual types. Cheek (1961) dealt with orgasmic dysfunction, claiming success in helping preorgasmic women by means of hypnosis. Wollman (1964) utilized hypnosis for sexual dysfunctions of both men and women, emphasizing imagery and mental rehearsal. Leckie (1964) employed hypnotic suggestions to relax patients with gynecological disorders. Schneck (1965) combined hypnotic relaxation with imagining to help women with vaginismus, as Dittborn (1957) had done before in treating erectile dysfunctions.

Others used hypnosis in conjunction with behavior therapy (Hussain, 1964), a combination which Lazarus (1973) found of therapeutic value. Many others, however, used hypnotic techniques without even mentioning hypnosis, as if they were not aware of the fact that their therapeutic method was hypnotic in nature. Under this category one can list all the authors who employed guided imagery, such as Wolpin (1969). Although the general principle of taking advantage of the human ability to imagine was comprehensively developed by Cautela (1967, 1970, 1971, 1977), his covert techniques have been used in behavior therapy generally, but not specifically in sex therapy.

Among the hypnotic methods using imagery and direct suggestions, I might cite the experimental work done by Cox and myself (Cox and Araoz, 1977) because in it we used very traditional hypnotic techniques, in order to validate the possible assistance to "persons who appear to be incapable of experiencing orgasm because of radical genital surgery, spinal cord damage or severe genital mutilation" (p. 83). The paper reported on three nondisabled women with whom such methods were employed. As we stated then:

> The results appear to justify optimism that it may be possible to restore orgasm to the disabled in concert with other rehabilitative measures. In addition to the benefit to the disabled, use of the same techniques could be effective in heightening the sexual responsiveness of the "normal" client and may provide a means of short-term treatment for sexual dysfunctions (p. 83).

If nondisabled women were able to experience orgasm without the presence of any normal sexual stimulus but merely through post-hypnotic suggestions (light touch of hand, light touch of forehead, counting by experimenter, counting by subject), it was hypothesized that the same hypnotic learning can take place in the disabled. Unfortunately, Cox and I did not have the opportunity to continue our work together and thus never tested our hypothesis with the disabled. Our experiment, however, imperfect as it was, seems to indicate that people can learn to experience orgasm. As we put it: "Since hypnosis has already proven to be an effective tool for increasing or decreasing a person's awareness of his/her body, it is natural to assume that it may be used to good avail in training clients to experience an orgasm" (p. 90).

This, indeed, is still my interest and contention: We can learn to use our mind in such a way that it can work *for* us. The association of hypnosis with sex therapy is the most parsimonious way to improve the human sexual experience.

THE PROFESSION OF SEX THERAPY

This historical review has thus far concentrated heavily on the contribution of "hypnotists." Of the three main authors examined, only Beigel was identified throughout his long career as a "sexologist," though his interest in hypnosis was there from the very beginning. Other popular authors, such as psychiatrist Caprio (see, e.g., Caprio and Berger, 1963) advocated hypnosis to improve one's sexual enjoyment, without a clear label of either sex therapist or hypnotist.

When we look into the field of sex therapy, we do not find the direct use of hypnosis, except in exceptional cases, as with Beigel. But, before going any further, we should remember that the so-called sex therapy "profession" is still a controversial issue, because of its very nature and its method of treatment. First, it is difficult to pinpoint the chronological origin of sex therapy. LoPiccolo (1978) wrote about "the quiet revolution in American psychotherapy" begun in the late 1950s with the emergence of short-term techniques based on learning theory and direct retraining of behavior in the here and now. This approach was used to help patients with all types of anxiety, one of them being sexual anxiety. As LoPiccolo stated,

Therapists such as Wolpe (1958), Hastings (1963) and Ellis (1966), in dealing with sexual problems, focused on various procedures such as reducing anxiety about sexual performance, changing negative attitudes towards sexuality, increasing communication between the couple and education and training in sexual physiology and sexual techniques (p. 513).

Later, in the 1970s, the interest in sex therapy grew tremendously and this specialization became formalized with the trappings of a "profession." Thus, training in sex therapy became fashionable; sex therapy institutes and programs proliferated, and the American Association of Sex Educators and Counselors added a new category, namely *Therapists*, to its name (A.A.S.E.C.T.) and formalized a "certification" procedure for sex therapists. Thus, the publication of *Human Sexual Response* by Masters and Johnson in 1966 signaled the beginning of sex therapy as a specialization, while A.A.S.E.C.T.'s certification of sex therapists, starting in 1974, may be considered the origin of the "profession" of sex therapy. These two historical landmarks deserve some attention.

MASTERS AND JOHNSON

The story is told that Masters and Johnson did not plan to publish in 1966 the results of their ten years of laboratory studies about human sexuality. The word that they were engaged in this type of research got out and, to avoid misunderstandings, they produced *Human Sexual Response,* a comprehensive report about the almost 600 men and women studied during over 2,500 sexual response cycles, addressed to the scientific community, not the general public. But since the interest in the topic was so great, soon the book became a bestseller in spite of the technical jargon in the detailed descriptions of sexual physiology and response during coitus and masturbation in people from 18 to 89 years of age.

Among the many important contributions of their first major work (1966), Masters and Johnson established the four stages of sexual response, namely, excitement, plateau, orgasm, and resolution. These define the anatomical and physiological differences between arousal and orgasm, known since as the *biphasic* nature of the human sexual response. Their main contribution was to systematize sex therapy as a functional combination of directive, educational, and behavioristic techniques.

The work of Masters and Johnson had been held in great esteem until Zilbergeld and Evans (1980) presented their criticism of *Human Sexual Inadequacy* (1970) and *Homosexuality in Perspective* (1979), the two latest major works by Masters and Johnson. Zilbergeld and Evans contend that the first book, *Human Sexual Response* (1966), was so well received that their two later works on treatment outcome benefited from a halo effect, since the evidence for all sex therapy is equivocal. In *Human Sexual Inadequacy*, for example, the data were presented in terms of a 20 percent failure rate, leading to the popular interpretation that Masters and Johnson were reporting on a 80 percent success rate, which is far from the truth.

Other serious flaws from a research point of view, according to Zilbergeld and Evans, affect the subjects, the procedure, and the follow-up. Regarding the subjects, the number and characteristics of the applicants rejected for treatment were not given. If only "good" clients were taken, the data would not reflect what happens in most clinical practices. Also, no mention was made of dropouts in the Masters and Johnson program. Regarding the procedure itself, the program was said to last two weeks but the number of contact hours this entails was not given. Since telephone contact was maintained after the two-week program was finished, one does not really know the exact length of the entire procedure. Finally, the follow-up data were based on incomplete information. Consequently, Zilbergeld and Evans question the long-term effectiveness of the program (7 percent relapse rate in the 1970 volume), especially when the data are compared with other sex therapists' results, with a relapse rate typically above 35 percent.

In *Homosexuality in Perspective*, the two critics found also many questions. The low (35 percent) failure rate, for instance, can be attributed only partly to the effectiveness of the treatment. Another major factor was the characteristics of the clients themselves who, Zilbergeld and Evans believe, were bisexuals or confused heterosexuals instead of true homosexuals, based on the screening methods used by Masters and Johnson. Furthermore, their treatment techniques were not reported in any meaningful detail.

Without questioning the critics' motivation, their comments cannot make us forget the undisputed greatness of Masters and Johnson's contributions to the field of human sexuality. Among their contributions, they exploded three myths that had been prevalent for many generations, namely, that of the importance of a large-sized penis in intercourse, that of vaginal orgasm, and the previously questioned capacity of the average woman for multiple orgasms in rapid succession.

They also opened up new paths for research on sexual behavior, objectifying an area of human activity which had escaped the direct observation of science. They also understood in a deeply humane way the emotional, interpersonal components of human sexuality, insisting on treating the sexual problem as a couple problem way before systems theory was popular in relational therapy. Finally, perhaps the major contribution of Masters and Johnson was their method of rapid treatment of sexual dysfunctions, focusing on the learning processes rather than on psychodynamic forces.

No criticism can take away these real contributions, but the flaws in important studies in this field remind us of the fact that sex therapy still has a long way to go in order to establish its theory and data in a solid fashion.

CERTIFICATION OF SEX THERAPISTS

The second historical event in the profession of sex therapy is the national certification of sex therapists by A.A.S.E.C.T., starting in 1974. Here, too, one finds more questions than answers. LoPiccolo (1978) examines the procedure carefully and concludes that, in spite of this certification, "quality controls are sadly lacking," because A.A.S.E.C.T. "has not been effective in guaranteeing the competence of the practitioners of sex therapy" (p. 524). The main reason for his statement lies in the fact that "A.A.S.E.C.T.'s standards for certification are probably too low to guarantee uniform competence" (p. 522), though he admits that many prestigious sex therapists have voluntarily submitted to this certification, perhaps because it is the only such program for the professional who wants to identify him/herself as an expert in sex therapy. The certification program, by the way, is interdisciplinary, including all mental health professionals.

If one of the most serious research studies in the field seems to be imperfect and the certification of sex therapists appears weak, one can hardly call this field an independent profession. In practice, moreover, most sex therapists also do other types of therapy, making sex therapy professionals a rather small number, while the mental health workers who practice sex therapy are, indeed, many.

HELEN SINGER KAPLAN

The second controversial issue about sex therapy as a profession concentrates on its very method of treatment, mostly from a theoretical point of view. Why should sex therapy occupy such a special place, when it is basically the application of behavior modification methods to sexual problems (Jehu, 1979)? If one considers the work of Masters and Johnson and of the "traditional" sex therapists who followed their approach, it is difficult, indeed, to answer the question satisfactorily. However, Kaplan (1979) has defined sex therapy as a unique method of therapy, different from both the psychoanalytical model and the behavioral one, calling it "psychosexual therapy." This uniqueness consists in her adept progress from (a) behavioristic interventions to (b) helping patients attain immediate awareness of patterns and causes, moving, when necessary, to (c) a deeper developmental insight—her "multicausal levels concept." Kaplan, therefore, building on Masters and Johnson and refining the method of therapy, gives an answer to those who object to sex therapy as a unique type of therapy. Already in her first book (1974) Kaplan mentioned a comprehensive approach in sex therapy—a progressive method from behavioral techniques to deep psychodynamics. In her own words:

> The sexual tasks are essential ingredients of sex therapy. However, I believe they are of limited value unless they are conducted within a rational psychotherapeutic context. On the other hand, by itself psychotherapy is a relatively ineffective or at best slow method of treating the sexual dysfunctions. However, when the two modalities are used in combination . . . psychotherapy . . . is indispensable to the success of the new sex therapy (p. 221).

Based on her thinking about sexual abulia (Kaplan, 1979) I have outlined a model for all psychogenic sexual dysfunctions. The figure shows sexual dysfunction as a process with antecedents and results at two levels, remote and immediate.

Figure

Remote Antecedent	Immediate Antecedent		Immediate Result	Remote Result
Psychogenic factors: faulty learning, negative experiences, etc.	Sexual anxiety (Negative self-hypnosis)		No libido *or* avoidance of sexual opportunities *or wrong sexual choices*	No sex *or* sexual "failure"

The immediate antecedent for sexual dysfunctions is anxiety, which is fed by the process of negative self-talk and defeatist imagery —what I have called negative self-hypnosis (Araoz, 1981a) and with which I shall deal later on. The important contribution made by Kaplan is her stress on "thinking" as crucial in sexual functioning. As I stated in the review of her book (Araoz, 1980c), "Sexual anxiety produces sexual antibodies, as it were, in the form of negativistic mental activities which inhibit sexual desire" (p. 84). These negative mental activities form what she designates as the "turn-off mechanism," mentioned previously. To repeat, sexual anxiety consists of a self-induced mental process which starts with a sexual stimulus (external or internal). This triggers either unpleasant memories of past failures and hurt or fears of imagined disappointments. The next step is the active involvement in negative self-talk, memories, images, myths, projections, and so on, which increases the anxiety and diminishes the desire for any type of sexual activity. This active mental exercise is mostly subconscious, though in many cases it eventually becomes quite conscious and deliberate.

Kaplan, therefore, focusing on sexual abulia, points to one of the most important elements to be considered in sex therapy, namely, the "thinking" of the patient—his/her cognitions. I shall develop these concepts in Chapter Four, but it is important to stress here that the systematic study of cognitions in human sexual behavior is attracting increasingly the attention of researchers and clinicians alike (see Rosen, Leiblum, and Gagnon, 1979).

LATEST DEVELOPMENTS IN SEX THERAPY

It can be seen that, though hypnosis as such is rarely used by sex therapists, the hypnotic phenomena of autosuggestion, negative self-talk, self-induced defeatist imagery, and the like are very much part of the current thinking in sex therapy, as I hope to show in the next few paragraphs. A review of papers on sex therapy and research published in 1980 alone gives us over 12 articles dealing with the hypnotic phenomena mentioned above. One of them is the very important paper by Mosher (1980) on the three dimensions of depth of involvement in human sexual response, which I will discuss in Chapter Four.

Three articles have been selected for more detailed review. These are of interest to the sex therapist because of the factual information they convey.

Sex and Imagery Ability

Harris, Yulis, and Lacoste (1980) investigated the relationship between sexual arousability and imagery ability and, again, between this mental ability and Eysenck's introversion personality dimension. Since sexual arousal can happen by a classical conditioning process (a particular food allegedly having sexual arousability properties), it seems reasonable to expect that those people who are able to form conditioned responses easily become sexually aroused by a larger number of situations than those who find it difficult to establish the connection between a neutral stimulus and a sexual response. Erotic imagery is considered a conditioned stimulus leading to sexual arousal, and, therefore, those people who are good at imagery formation would be expected to become sexually aroused more highly and more and more often than those whose imagery ability is poor.

Using Hoon, Hoon, and Wincze's (1976) *Sexual Arousability Inventory* (SAI), Harris et al. measured sexual arousal. To measure conditionability, *Eysenck's Personality Inventory: Form A* (EPI) (Eysenck and Eysenck, 1963) was used, since, according to its findings, introverts form conditioned responses more easily than extra-verts. The authors' prediction was that introverts, when compared to extraverts, would report forming more vivid images. Finally, to meas-ure imagery ability, the *Betts Questionnaire Upon Mental Imagery (Short Form)* (Sheehan, 1967) was employed. The authors recruited 100 males and 100 females from among undergraduate students from 18 to 25 years of age. The EPI, BETTS, and SAI were adminis-tered to each volunteer in one sitting, lasting about 20 minutes. The results confirmed that imagery ability was associated with higher sexu-al arousal, justifying the clinical use of imagination to enhance sexual response in sexually dysfunctional patients. On the other hand, the findings of this study indicate that conditionability and imagery ability are *not related*. It is also interesting to note that there was a difference between males and females. For the latter, the personality scores were helpful in predicting the sexual arousal scores, whereas for males this was not the case.

Harris, Yulis, and Lacoste insisted on "clear, vivid images," which are only possible when the person enters an alternate state of aware-ness—the experience of hypnosis—leaving aside the critical, logical, mental functions. Their carefully conducted study confirmed my con-tention that hypnosis is the method of choice to deal with sexual dysfunctions of a psychogenic origin, and also validated the generally accepted notion that imagery is a regular concomitant of human sex-ual behavior in all its phases.

Sexual Arousal Through Imagery

The second study I chose to review as a sample of the latest thinking in sex therapy was conducted by Mosher and White (1980) with 100 college females who listened to erotic guided imagery and then report-ed on their sexual arousal and on ten emotions, ranging from anger and contempt to interest and enjoyment. However, the main thrust of this study was to research the effects of either *causal* or *committed* sexual imagery on young females' arousal and emotions. Mosher and White used six measures: (a) a guilty inventory; (b) a heterosexual be-havior assessment; (c) a rating of sexual arousal; (d) a self-report of genital sensations; (e) an effective sexual arousal scale; and (f) a differential emotions scale measuring ten emotions related to sexual arousal.

The experimental session was arranged so that 64 women participated in the casual sex imagery scenarios and 36 in the commited condition. A tape recording of a woman's voice started by inviting the subjects to relax and then proceeded to present guided imagery of a sexual invitation. This was followed by the volunteers' assessment of their sexual arousal and their emotional experience. Immediately thereafter, the same voice suggested relaxation once more and then presented imagery of sexual intercourse. Again, the subjects were asked to evaluate the latter experience as before. After the second subjective assessment, the taped female voice invited the subjects to relax for the third time and then continued by presenting "guided imagery of a retrospective reflection on the meaning and significance of the sexual experience" (p. 280). Then, for the third time, the subjects evaluated the latter part, as before. Finally, the volunteers were relaxed one last time before ending the experiment.

The results of this research emphasize items related to committed or casual sex. However, the authors' use of guided imagery with relaxation—definitely hypnotic techniques—confirms the usefulness of this method, with implications for clinical work. This research, which won an award from the Society for the Scientific Study of Sex, is indicative of the current interest in hypnotic methods in the field of sex therapy. Mosher and White finished their report by suggesting new uses of what they call guided imagery techniques for both sex research and therapy. As I have discussed in Chapter One, successful guided imagery is, indeed, hypnosis.

Cognition and Sex

Based on a thoughtful review of the evidence gathered from many studies, Walen (1980) proposes a new conception of the sexual arousal cycle, emphasizing the cognitive elements involved in human sexuality. As she states: "This system suggests a feedback model in which each of the eight links in the chain functions as both a cue for the next link and a reinforcer for the preceding event" (p. 89). The eight links are: (1) perception of a sexual stimulus; (2) evaluation of the stimulus;

(3) physiological arousal; (4) perception of the arousal; (5) evaluation of the arousal and its perception; (6) sexual behavior; (7) perception of that behavior; and (8) evaluation of the sexual behavior. It should be noted that links 1, 2, 4, 5, 7, and 8 are purely cognitive operations and hypnotic in nature, since they are in Walen's description eminently *subjective* perceptions and evaluations.

The evidence on which Walen builds this new theory of sexual behavior is quite solid, although she herself did not conduct a particular study before presenting her data. She constructs her theory on two elements of cognitive therapy, namely, perception and evaluation. Then, she gathers evidence from other researchers who have conducted studies on human sexuality both clinically and experimentally and uses their data to validate her theoretical formulation. In her words, "Positive sexual experiences are a smooth amalgam of stimuli and responses, the flow between them guided by correct perceptions and positive evaluations" (p. 95). These perceptions and evaluations are mostly subconscious, outside the area of reason and logic, and, consequently, hypnotic in nature.

Walen notes that the traditional categories of sexual dysfunctions (ejaculatory and erectile dysfunctions for men, and preorgasmia, dyspareunia, and vaginismus among women) have as a common element the same dysfunctional cognitive processes of incorrect or negative cognitions. As she states: "It appears that the core ingredients in all of the diagnostic categories are a high level of emotional distress induced by cognitive errors of evaluation, often coupled with cognitive errors of perception. The end product is an individual who approaches the job of sex (rather than the joy of sex) as a way to prove him/herself (rather than to enjoy him/herself) —certainly a very unsexy attitude" (p. 96). Rather than focusing on specific sexual behaviors, she suggests that sex therapy concern itself more directly with the emotional disturbance and the nonplayful attitudes of the individual, since these two cognitive factors become direct impediments to sexual enjoyment.

Walen's paper is an important theoretical contribution to sex therapy, and the fact that it was published in one of the prestigious sex therapy journals is another indication of the increased awareness of and current interest in the ways the human mind influences sexual behavior and, consequently, the urgent need of sex therapy to transcend sex technique. All the "sexpertise" in the world cannot overcome "inhibitions, guilt, anxiety, depression or anger." Walen seems to accept Kaplan's (1979) challenge to move from sex therapy to "psychosexual therapy."

CONCLUSION

Concluding this section on sex therapy, it can be said that, *if hypnosis is the experience of focused concentration with minimal critical, logical, sequential mental activity* (as Chapter One discussed in detail), *then we see that sex therapy, especially in the last few years, is using hypnosis as an important element in its clinical approach.* From the very beginning of sex therapy, as distinct from other types of therapy, one finds "hypnotic" elements. However, even at present these hypnotic elements have not been developed systematically. In general, there seems to be a reluctance among sex therapists to employ hypnosis—or, at least, to admit openly to the use of hypnosis. It may also be that those sex therapists who are engaged in hypnosis in their work are not fully aware that what they are doing is, indeed, hypnosis. This may come from the common misunderstanding that hypnosis is still fixed in the traditional, ritualistic method with which most professionals are vaguely acquainted. In explaining The New Hypnosis in Chapter One, I have attempted to show that the techniques reviewed in the last sections of this chapter are, truly, hypnosis.

This second chapter addressed itself to the historical foundations for the integration of hypnosis and sex therapy. The review of the evidence for such integration started with authors and clinicians who must be identified as *hypnotherapists,* as opposed to *sex therapists.* But, even here, Beigel is an important figure in the latter field. Then I presented significant evidence of hypnotic methods used in sex therapy as such.

Among the former group, I found indirect imagination methods, as represented by Erickson, uncovering and suggestion methods, exemplified by van Pelt, and exploration and *in vivo* rehearsal methods, as advocated by Beigel. However, besides these three main approaches, the literature presents direct suggestion methods, though mostly heavily depending on imagery. From this review, it seems fair to conclude that the combination of hypnosis and sex therapy is not only a useful clinical method but apparently the most parsimonious way to improve the human sexual experience—the latter being the goal of sex therapy.

Then, my investigation moved to the field of sex therapy proper. Although Masters and Johnson had hinted at the area of cognition and imagination in sexual behavior, they did not develop either the theory to understand these elements or the techniques to deal with them. Almost a decade later, Kaplan came much closer to the area of hypnosis (cognition and imagination) in human sexuality but, again, fell short of the mark. Later developments in sex therapy research and application do focus more specifically on hypnotic methods, as my review of studies published in 1980 indicates.

The historical developments in both fields warrant, therefore, my attempt at integrating the contributions from both. This attempted integration will enrich our understanding of human sexuality, on the one hand, and of the cognitive/imaginative processes in human functioning in general and in sexual behavior in particular, on the other.

To conclude this chapter, mention should be made again of the interesting paper first presented at the annual meeting of the American Psychological Association in 1978 and then published in the Spring of 1980. Its title is self-explanatory, namely, "Hypnosis in the Treatment of Sexual Dysfunction" (Brown and Chaves, 1980). The conclusions of the authors are that more controlled studies to ascertain the efficacy of hypnosis in treating sexual dysfunctions are needed. I am in full agreement with this statement, though, as Brown and Chaves state, "the hypnotherapy of sexual dysfunction is not an easy area in which to do research" (p. 73). However, let us note that in no way do the authors discredit the notion of using hypnosis in sex therapy. On the contrary, they encourage its use, though with the caution of being more careful so that valid data can be obtained.

The historical development of the use of hypnosis in sex therapy shows that we are now at a propitious time to attempt to integrate both fields. The next chapters will deal with the theoretical foundations for using hypnosis in sex therapy. I will examine this area from different angles, namely, those of cognitive therapy, sex research, and hypnosis research.

3

Theoretical background

The theory for applying hypnosis in sex therapy is merely an aspect of the theory behind cognitive (behavior) therapy. Contrary to Steger (1978), I stress that hypnosis is a method of cognitive restructuring and thus can fall within a cognitive (behavioral) frame of reference. In my understanding of hypnosis (Chapter One), true cognitive modification implies hypnotic processes and techniques.

COGNITIVE (BEHAVIOR) THERAPY

It must be stated from the outset that, unlike some cognitive behavior therapy authors, I consider *cognitions* to encompass all mental activities involved in perception, evaluation, and interpretation of stimuli, both internal and external. This includes subconscious as well as conscious mental activiies. To me, *cognition* is a modern expression for the old term, *mentation,* found frequently in early 20th century psychologists' works. Therefore, cognitions are beliefs and ideas but also mental images, i.e., mental representations of sensory experiences replicating the external senses through which we perceive (see the section in this chapter on Mental Images or Mental Pictures?). Cognitive restructuring is meaningless without including those other "cognitions" less ideological and intellectual, such as mental imagery.

In the same vein, I refer to "thinking"—usually in quotes—to indicate any form of mental activity, including "spontaneous thinking" such as daydreaming, fantasy, and any mental representational system activated consciously or not in the individual. It should also be remembered that *mind* is a catch-all word to indicate even the most subtle and unknown functions of the human *brain*.

The roots of the rather recent emphasis on cognitions in therapy go deep into behavior therapy proper and beyond. Epictetus, a Greek Stoic of the first century A.D., who taught in Rome, is quoted often as stating that "Men are disturbed not by things but by the view which they have of them." Similarly, the "Eightfold Path" of the Buddha could be translated into cognitive self-control prescriptions (Rahula, 1959).

Among the best proponents of cognitive therapy are Beck (1976) and Meichenbaum (1977). Before one studies them, a brief digression into behavior therapy is useful. As others have pointed out (Romanczyk and Kistner, 1977; Wilson, 1978a), it is necessary to make a distinction between *operant behavior modification*, with Skinner (1953, 1971) as a leader, and Eysenck's (1960, 1964) and Wolpe's (1958) *behavior therapy,* which follows the classical conditioning model. Besides these two forms of behavioral interventions, Bandura's (1969) *social-learning model* in behavior therapy is a comprehensive approach to human functioning including (1) external stimulus events, following classical conditioning processes; (2) external reinforcement or operant conditioning at work; and (3) *cognitive mediational processes,* which are the all-important factors in behavior modification through the influence of environmental events. It is *easy* to see that the latter model of behavior therapy is almost diametrically opposed to Skinner's (1971) famous statement: "A person does not act upon the world; the world acts upon him" (p. 211).

The social-learning theory of behavior therapy, therefore, prepares the ground for the development of cognitive (behavior) therapy. The distinction between these two theories is beyond the scope of my discussion and the reader is referred to Franks and Wilson (1973-1979). I prefer to write the word *behavior* in parenthesis to stress that the changes in "thinking" are the essentials of this therapeutic approach and to deemphasize the types of behavior therapy of both Skinner and Wolpe. Moreover, behavior should be the ultimate concern in all therapies, including psychoanalysis.

To return now to the two authors mentioned earlier, it would be theoretically and historically inaccurate to center cognitive therapy around Beck (1976) and Meichenbaum (1977) without referring to Ellis (1962), whose Rational Emotive Therapy (RET) influenced them, and who must be considered one of the major forces in cognitive therapy. Indeed, RET is the oldest cognitive therapy and perhaps most popular and well-known among professionals and laymen alike. For more than two decades, Ellis has influenced clinical psychology, and even the American public in general, through many self-help books which have borrowed heavily from his teachings. Cognitive therapy is another example of Ellis' influence: Both Beck's (1976) approach and Meichenbaum's (1973) self-instructional training (SIT) are really variations of RET. Lazarus (1976), another important author very influenced by Ellis, was one of the first behavior therapists to apply primarily cognitive techniques (Lazarus, 1971), considering self-talk and mental imagery essential factors to keep in mind in any form of attempted behavior change.

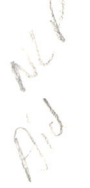

As I have stated elsewhere (Araoz, 1981a), the techniques of cognitive therapy are basically hypnotic in nature. Moreover, the rationale for the cognitive approaches is the reality of the patient's negative self-hypnosis. What Ellis calls *irrational* beliefs are really one aspect of what I have identified as *negative self-hypnosis*. This process seems to be present in all people who find themselves fixated in behaviors, attitudes, beliefs, fears, reactions, patterns, drives, goals, thoughts, and loves with which they are dissatisfied. Negative self-hypnosis (NSH) seems to be the common denominator of psychogenic problems.

What is this mental process I call NSH? It consists of the nonconscious negative statements and defeatist mental images that a person indulges in, encourages, and, often, even works hard at fostering, while, at the same time, consciously saying to him/herself that s/he wants to solve the problem, wants to change, wants to get better. As long as NSH is at work, no improvement is possible. But why call this mental process NSH? Because in it we find three hypnotic elements included in any serious understanding of hypnosis: (1) noncritical thinking which becomes a negative activation of subconscious processes; (2) active negative imagery; and (3) powerful posthypnotic suggestions in the form of negative self-affirmations coming from the non-critical thinking and the negative imagery.

I should add that NSH is not exactly what psychoanalysis calls resistance and what practically every other method of therapy since Freud has incorporated in its conceptualization. NSH is closest to what Kris(1956) called the *resistant structure*. Resistance, as it is used commonly, has to do with the use of defense mechanisms in the psychoanalytic session. NSH is not necessarily rooted in anxiety or conflict, as the mechanisms of defense are, but it may have its origins in cultural myths, false pseudo-religious beliefs, and folk superstition. NSH is much more hypnotic than resistance, as its definition suggests; however, obviously, it can be part of the resistant structure in therapy itself or of the exaggerated use of defense mechanisms in general.

In the following example, there is a resistance to change, but it is rooted in deeper levels affecting the self-concept than defense mechanisms are. The person who says, "I cannot do what I know I should do,' referring to breaking up a damaging relationship affecting the person's sexual behavior, is really unable to change because s/he is *convinced* that s/he cannot end that relationship. That conviction is the result of a negative self-hypnotic process, consisting of self-talk convincing him/herself that this breakup is impossible and fostering, perhaps even actively fomenting, all sorts of mental images of horror and catastrophe connected with the breakup. Through this repetitive process, his/her subconscious has come to accept non-critically that ending this relationship is quite impossible. Perceptions have been distorted, evaluations are wrong, change cannot take place, the cycle of misery is strengthened.

What cognitive therapy intends to do is to counteract NSH. Meichenbaum (1973), basing his therapeutic approach on the research of the developmental sequence followed by children in learning internal speech and verbal-symbolic control over their behavior (see Luria, 1961), proposes his by now famous self-instructional training. The procedure comprises three basic steps: (a) identification and awareness of one's maladaptive thoughts manifested in negative self-statements; (b) learning of appropriate behaviors and positive self-statements; and (c) practice, first while verbalizing aloud the appropriate self-instructions and later by *rehearsing them in fantasy*. During this phase of therapy, the therapist gives feedback to ensure that *positive self-talk* replaces the previously identified negative self-statements. Although up to this point we have conscious restructuring of cognitions, the last step, emphasizing covert or imaginary rehearsal, leads naturally into a subconscious process, slowly becoming a new attitude that has all the elements of a post-hypnotic suggestion. Several studies conducted by Meichenbaum (1974; Meichenbaum and Cameron, 1973) demonstrate the effectiveness of this method.

Beck (1976) employs basically the same approach, combining behavioral and cognitive techniques with emphasis on home practice. Slightly different modalities of these methods have been used by Kazdin (1974) under the name of *covert modeling,* by Suinn and Richardson (1971) *(anxiety-management training),* by Goldfried (1971) *(modified systematic desensitization),* and others. They all use imagination or covert conditioning. Perhaps the best exponent of covert techniques is Cautela (1966, 1967, 1970, 1971). He defines this method as "Conditioning procedures in which the stimuli and responses are presented in imagination via instructions" (Cautela, 1975). He explains that covert conditioning has similar effects on behavior to external stimuli, as controlled studies have proven. The four primary techniques of covert conditioning are sensitization, positive reinforcement, negative reinforcement, and extinction.

There is no question that behavior therapy "has gone cognitive," which means that more and more emphasis is placed nowadays on the activities of the *organism* (O) in between the stimulus and the response. Wolpe and Skinner, as was mentioned earlier, stressed the S-R model of human behavior, while the current trend emphasizes the S-O-R model, paying close attention to the mediating structures and processes between S and R, since accumulated evidence shows that there is no S without O—in other words, that the stimulus, if it does not impinge on the organism, is an indifferent entity.

For further evidence of the definite emphasis on "thinking" in current psychotherapy approaches, the reader is directed to *Cognitive Therapy and Research,* a journal started in 1977.

THE HYPNOBEHAVIORAL MODEL

From the field of hypnotherapy proper, Kroger and Fezler (1976) developed an elegant model, in part based on the Hypno-Operant Therapy of Tugender and Ferinden (1972). "The basic premise in the hypnobehavioral model is that maladaptive responses are anxiety mediated" (Kroger and Fezler, 1976, p. 91). To remedy this situation, the authors employ *hypnorelaxation*, since they see it as the antithesis of anxiety and tension. Their definition of hypnosis is: "A state of profound relaxation and concentration by means of sensory recall characterized by increased receptivity and objectivity" (pp. 86 and 89). By objectivity they seem to mean that the person using hypnosis is more able to take action without interference of subjective anxiety and fear. They claim that the use of hypnosis "strengthens the standard covert desensitization models used by the behavior modifiers" (p. 86-87) and refer to the studies of the Russian researcher Platonov (1959) to validate their claim that "conditioning of reflexes under hypnosis is more durable, rapid and less likely to extinguish" (p. 87). This greater efficacy of hypnotic methods is empathically attributed by Kroger and Fezler to sensory recall or imagery conditioning:

> Being able to induce relaxation through sensory imagery gives the patient far more control than resorting to direct muscular manipulation as employed by Jacobson's progressive relaxation techniques. Also, a much deeper state of relaxation can be achieved through sensory recall than through direct muscle manipulation. Both hypnosis and standard behavior modification make use of sensory imagery conditioning, but the former results in more control even over much autonomic functioning (p. 90).

The hypnobehavioral model is a clever combination of hypnosis with behavior modification. It would be hard to find the real difference between Kroger and Fezler's model and many of the techniques mentioned in the previous section, especially those employed by Cautela under the rubric of *covert* procedures. The more one emphasizes the covert aspect of the procedure, the more hypnosis is used. As I explained in Chapter One, hypnosis is not an all or nothing experience. The difficult question to answer, from an experimental point of view, is posed by very ordinary experiences of everyday living, that is: At what point does sensory recall or active imagining become hypnosis? Or, more to the point of therapy: At what point—whether the therapist thinks of it or not, whether s/he realizes what s/he is doing or not—do covert techniques become hypnosis? As Kroger and

Fezler imply and as I have stressed, based on the data provided by reputable research, hypnosis is a skill that can be learned through repetition and practice. Consequently, the more intense are the covert techniques and the more vivid are the sensory recall and the imagery production, the more the person is using hypnosis. Or, to put this thought in Kroger and Fezler's own words: "The combination of behavior therapy and hypnosis provides the clinician with a wide variety of sophisticated and more powerful techniques for treating problems refractory to conventional psychotherapies" (p. 95).

These authors apply their model of hypnobehavioral therapy to a variety of sexual dysfunctions, in line with the current thinking about effective change in the human condition, as mentioned earlier in this chapter.

SEX THERAPY

In a special issue of *The Counseling Psychologist* (1975), two important articles were published which signal a turning point in sex therapy—the beginning of an emphasis on imagery techniques as opposed to the purely or primarily behavioral emphasis in sex therapy. Wish (1975) started with Masters and Johnson's work to justify the use of techniques to reach the cognitive processes of the clients who are sexually dysfunctional. Then he considered Kaplan's goal of helping people abandon themselves completely to the sexual experience and her desire to minimize the internally reinforced performance anxiety. From the writings of these major contributors in sex therapy, Wish concluded that, "Whatever the treatment given, the goal is to enable the dysfunctional client to relax and focus attention on incoming erotic stimuli" (p. 52). Then he proposed a series of techniques, such as thought stopping, covert assertion and conditioning, and systematic desensitization, based on the general principles of cognitive therapy. As Wish summarized it: "Theoretical and empirical support lies in the fact that covert events share many of the same functional properties known to exist for overt behavior and, therefore, by manipulating covert processes one can modify overt consequences" (p. 52). The sources he used are those of behavior therapy, such as Bandura (1969), Cautela, Walsh and Wish (1971), Pavio (1969), and Staas (1972).

Another study by Flowers and Booraem (1975) observed the behavior of three different but related client groups in sex therapy, i.e.: "(1) those who resist initial behavioral interventions because of anxiety or on moral grounds; (2) those who engage in initial behavioral interventions and experience failure, often associated with failure fantasies; and (3) those who succeed technically at behavioral interventions but fail to reach the desired level of excitation" (p. 50). They found a deficit of sexual fantasy in these clients and through visualization training, as a first step, claim to have obtained encouraging success.

I cite this study because it confirms the theoretical principle mentioned above, which gives scientific validation to the old aphorism, "As a man thinketh in his heart, so is he." Flowers and Booraem provide us with data for the theoretical position advanced thus far, namely, that behavior can change by use of imagery geared to the changes desired. To me it is interesting to note that the scientific facts that we are accumulating simply confirm what has been held to be true for many generations. I found a poem—exact date unknown—attributed to someone living in the 17th century, which is curiously pertinent to the theoretical justification for concentrating on "thinking" in order to improve "actions."

Mind is the Master-power that moulds and makes,
And Man is Mind, and evermore he takes
The tool of Thought, and, shaping what he wills,
Brings forth a thousand joys, a thousand ills: —
He thinks in secret and it comes to pass:
Environment is but his looking-glass. (my emphasis).

Still in the field of sex therapy as such, Janda and O'Grady (1980) developed a sex anxiety inventory which, used together with Mosher's (1965, 1966) guilt inventory, "could predict sexual behavior more accurately than either used alone" (p. 170). Janda and O'Grady make an interesting distinction between guilt and anxiety when it comes to sexual behavior: "The guilty individuals are concerned with what they will think of themselves, whereas sexually anxious individuals are concerned with what others will think of them" (p. 170).

The point in mentioning Janda and O'Grady's sexual anxiety inventory is their theoretical justification for having engaged in such an important and careful study, i.e., the negative attitudes and emotions towards sex of which current research is becoming increasingly aware. Negative attitudes and emotions are other terms for cognitions. Because Janda and O'Grady recognize that negative cognitions must be altered before any success is expected from sex therapy, they developed the sex anxiety inventory. This, together with Mosher's sex guilt inventory, helps the clinician identify the negative cognitions making sexual behavior dysfunctional and dissatisfying to the individual. The theoretical structure behind their research is in agreement with what I have investigated in this chapter.

We have noted that in cognitive therapy imagination occupies a very important place. When cognitive therapists explain what they mean by cognitions, they universally, in one way or another, include imagery. We can say that the evidence shows that *behind every sexual dysfunction lies a defective cognition*—negative affirmations and defeatist imagery—often not fully recognized by the sexually dysfunctional individual. The therapeutic approaches developed in the last decade or so aim at counteracting those negative cognitions and substitute effective thoughts—positive affirmations and constructive imagery—to make the previous cognitions inoperative. Hypnosis, as it is presently understood, constitutes a systematic use of cognitions for the improvement of the sexually dysfunctional individual.

As indicated before, in a true sense The New Hypnosis is a descendant of the Nancy school of hypnosis, where Bernheim (1964) claimed in the late 1880s that hypnosis was the effect of suggestion and defined suggestibility as the ability to transform a thought into an act. Emile Coué (1922), the originator of the term "autosuggestion," mentioned the power of positive imagery, as well as of verbal statements. His famous slogan, "Every day in every way I am getting better and better," was to be accompanied by vivid imagery of the desired behavior or improvement.

WHY DOES IMAGERY LEAD TO CHANGE?

On the basis of the investigation conducted so far, we may state that the principles of cognitive therapy underlie the current interest in the effects of "thinking" on sexual behavior and enjoyment. We still must ask: Why does imagery have such an effect on behavior? As Singer and Pope (1978) state, psychology, at least through more than half of this century, gave little heed to imagination in its research. Meichenbaum (1978), on the other hand, indicates that one could conservatively list 20 ways in which imagination has been used in psychotherapy in the last few years. Because of the plethora of imagery procedures, he undertakes the task of searching for common elements in all these imagination techniques and examining imagery fits within the larger context of psychotherapy.

In an earlier work, Meichenbaum (1977) described in detail the three steps which explain behavioral change in any form of therapy. Briefly, these are (a) self-awareness, (b) new adaptive thoughts and images, and (c) *in vivo* practice. By self-awareness, he means a new perception of symptoms, the circumstances around them (both internal and external), and behaviors. The client becomes conscious of his/her internal dialogue about his/her problems. This is what Meichenbaum calls the beginning of the "translation process," intimately connected with the conceptualizations about the problems. By "translation" he means the progressive change in perception and evaluation regarding the presenting problem.

The second step in the process of change through psychotherapy is the development of new adaptive cognitions—thoughts and images. The new cognitions must initiate a new behavioral chain, incompatible with the maladaptive behaviors. Thus, habitual acts are now mediated by deliberate new cognitions that deautomatize those acts. This forced cognitive mediation is essential to behavioral change.

Finally, Meichenbaum's analysis shows that in any effective psychotherapy there is a last step of *in vivo* practice of the new behaviors, which are the outcome of the new adaptive self-talk and imagery.

Turning again to our original question—Why does imagery affect behavior?—he finds three psychological processes which explain why imagery-based therapies contribute to change. These three psychological processes are self-control, new meaning, and mental rehearsal. While reading Meichenbaum's explanation, it is useful to keep The New Hypnosis in mind; the merits he finds in "imagery-based therapies" are those which clinical hypnosis has claimed for itself, independently of the new cognitive therapies.

The first psychological process explaining the effectiveness of imagery in behavior change is "the sense of control that the client develops because of the monitoring and rehearsing of various images both in therapy and *in vivo*" (Meichenbaum, 1978, p. 392). Although "it is a mistake to infer the causative role of particular images in psychopathology without exploring their occurrence in 'normal' populations" (p. 388), the belief shared by both therapist and client that these spontaneous images affect moods and behaviors is of therapeutic value. The value lies in the client's new perception and conceptualization of his/her problems as involving his/her "thinking," specifically his/her mental images.

What we don't know is whether frightening and destructive cognitions lead *always* to maladaptive behavior. They may lead to adaptive planning in "normal" populations. But what we do know is that those negative "thoughts" are definitely unwelcome to clients, who often feel they cannot do anything about them. These "thoughts," moreover, create more discomfort, fear, depression, or other inner experiences for which therapy is sought. The emphasis on images teaches clients that they can control their "thoughts," and that their control will make a difference in their mood, perception of others, even in their physiological reactions. Self-control of mental images is a common trait of all the therapies which underscore imagery. By controlling mental images, the client learns also to alter his/her reaction to the formerly feared thoughts—in terms of both self-talk and of actions taken.

The second psychological process proposed by Meichenbaum to explain the efficacy of mental images for change is "the changed meaning or altered internal dialogue that precedes, accompanies, and follows instances of maladaptive behavior" (1978, p. 392). This is a natural consequence of the increased self-control through imagery. Successful control of images and self-talk leads to new perceptions of one's inner processes. And since perception precedes and determines meaning in general, the client who, at least in part, attributed his/her maladaptive behavior to his/her thoughts understands the whole situation differently and more hopefully.

Moreover, since the problem is not so much the negative thoughts but the client's reaction to them, s/he now has at his/her disposal new coping mechanisms to deal with the negative, destructive thoughts and images and consequently sees them differently—as an experience s/he has to learn to handle, not as one in which s/he is the victim. As Meichenbaum puts it: "Each time we ask our clients to engage in certain imagery exercises, we are also affecting his internal dialogue, what he says to himself about the image, the meaning system surrounding the image and his maladaptive behaviors" (1978, p. 390). When the client's imagery is changed, his/her internal self-talk is also changed; what s/he says to him/herself alters the meaning of the experience itself. Perhaps an example could help: Names not only describe but give meaning to things and situations, to people and events—the same sexual act is *disgusting* to one and *fun* to the next person.

The third and final psychological process which helps us understand why imagery affects behavior is "the mental rehearsal of behavioral alternatives that contribute to the development of coping skills" (Meichenbaum, 1978, p. 392). This mental preparation for diverse situations is the natural outcome of the two previous processes: The new conviction of self-control in the management of "thinking" (which makes the person perceive and understand the whole situation differently) leads to a mental rehearsal of fresh and novel ways of dealing with different situations. Meichenbaum warns against the mistake of proposing a *mastery* model, rather than a *coping* model, for clients. The mastery model encourages a mental rehearsal of perfect performance, while the coping model includes apprehension, mistakes, shortcomings, but copes with these, thus familiarizing the client with the necessary coping strategies—new thoughts and images—for handling difficulties and obstacles.

Thus, Meichenbaum gives us at least the general direction in which to go for the answer to the crucial question regarding the connection of imagery and behavior. The whole area still requires careful study; on the other hand, the concern about data and controlled evidence should not blind us to what common sense has told countless generations before us, namely, that thoughts tend to materialize into actions. Philosophers, religious leaders, and poets alike have been giving us this message for many generations. Popular writers have become rich selling this idea—from how to become rich by thinking rich to how to improve one's sexual enjoyment by using one's imagination. Our scientific concern should encourage us to find factual validation of this ageless belief without making us forget that it has been ingrained in humans.

MENTAL IMAGES OR MENTAL PICTURES?

Our theoretical review has presented us over and over again with the notion of mental imagery. However, this concept in itself is not as self-evident as it may seem. *Imago,* in Latin, is primarily a reproduction of something else and thus it is an active, energetic word. The emphasis is on reproducing, not on the image. That mental imagery does not mean only pictorial representations of our existential experiences is not at all clear in much of the literature. An otherwise interesting article (Wilkins, 1974) studying therapeutic imagery, just to cite one example, falls short of its mark by limiting imagery to mental pictures. But imagery comprises every and all mental re-presentation of stimuli capable of being perceived by our receptors. Bandler and Grinder (1975a, b) have popularized the notion of *inner representational systems,* referring to our mental ability to reproduce ideologically, in our mind, "sensations" or experiences had or capable of being had in our sense. Thus, it is convenient to refer to our *inner senses* and to conceive of our mind as capable of reproducing gustatory, olfactory, kinesthetic, and auditory, as well as visual, sensations.

It may be true, as we can ascertain empirically, that each person has a preferred representational system, so that some people are more adept at "visualizing" while others can reproduce internally sounds and music and still others can reexperience bodily sensations, and so on. However, because of what Bandler and Grinder (1975a) call the neurological, social, and individual constraints, we can never represent or reproduce the external world as it really exists. We always misrepresent the world to ourselves, so that "there is a necessary difference between the world and any particular model or representation of the world" (pp. 7-8). The authors use "model" to mean what I want to convey by the term "image." This mental representation of the world (image or model) involves three processes which necessarily make our perception of the world different from the world itself.

Bandler and Grinder (1975a) refer to this perceptual transformation in terms of generalization, deletion, and distortion. These three processes create for each one of us "rules" by which we behave and relate to our environment. Thus, *generalization* "is the process by which elements or pieces of a person's model become detached from their original experience and come to represent the entire category of which the experience is an example" (p. 14). An instance of this, according to the authors, is being burned when touching a hot stove. *Deletion* refers to the "process by which we selectively pay attention to certain dimensions of our experience and exclude others" (p. 15). They give as an example the ability humans have to cut off the sounds of many conversations in a meeting room in order to pay attention to what one single person is saying. Finally, *distortion* is "the process which allows us to make shifts in our experience of sensory data" (p. 16) as we do through imagination and fantasy. A good example of this is the artist's rendering of a landscape, modified by his/her own perception, far different from a photo picture of the same scene.

Our mental "images," therefore, are not necessarily either mental pictures or exact reproductions of the outside reality. We may apply these concepts to human sexuality. The all-important factor in human sexual behavior is the way sex is perceived by the individual through these processes of generalization, deletion, and distortion. The same three processes which are beneficial in helping us relate to the world and understand it can , if exaggerated, disfigure reality to the point of complete deformity. Thus, a man may have become convinced that all women are a threat to his being (generalization, distortion, and a deletion of his own experience with some women in his life who were kind, helpful, and good). Unless the therapist is aware of this complex mechanism of mental images, the traditional approach of sex therapy will be ineffective in changing the "cognitive" mechanisms of the client. As Bandler and Grinder (1975a) explain, the mental model of the client frequently impoverishes his/her experience. Since hypnosis makes possible concentration on one thing to the exclusion of others, it becomes a convenient tool for helping clients change or enrich their mental "models," allowing them to stop the overgeneralization, overdistortion, and overdeletion processes.

IMAGERY AND SYMBOLISM

Without becoming involved in philosophical controversy, we can attest from our daily experience that mental imagery is functional and essential in our ordinary behavior. Shorr (1977) gives a simple example: In approaching a red traffic light when driving someone seriously ill to a hospital, our imagination produces different possibilities—going through the red light and having an accident, or injuring a pedestrian, or being stopped by a police officer. On the other hand, we "see" our arriving a few seconds earlier to the hospital and thus perhaps saving a human life. Shorr concludes that the valuable function of imagery is to "provide a method by which alternatives can be tested without undergoing all the dangers involved" (p. 32). The same mechanism allows us to test in our mind possibilities of behaviors that are less urgent or dramatic than the one described.

Imagery, therefore, is a basically human trait. In fact, it may be one of the most human characteristics, as art—the materialization of mental images—amply demonstrates. Because humans can imagine, visualize, "dream," we produce the marvels that other species do not. Art has reality as a referent, at least remotely or tenuously. But this creative distortion of reality which is art points to the human ability—indeed, necessity—to produce symbols. We are all artists because we all abstract—abstraction being a normal process in thinking; abstraction being essential to deal with reality as we perceive it; abstraction being one element in imagery formation. But to abstract is to produce symbols, because our abstractions are our attempts to give meaning to our experiences, to make sense of what we experience both through our sensory receptors and within ourselves.

Perhaps it was Descartes (1596-1650), with his great influence on Western thought, who created the confusion regarding the unitary or holistic nature of humans. His dichotomy between physical and spiritual realities, linked only through God's action, is still very much with us, as, for instance, a look at 20th century Western medicine makes clear. Body is conceptualized as independent of mind and vice versa. Or else, distorting the Cartesian premise, mind was simply equated with brain. The reader is referred to Barbara Brown's (1980) magnificent work for further elucidation of these concepts.

The point I want to emphasize is that humans are almost compulsive in giving meaning—or trying to give meaning—to their perceptions. In the process, they create symbols—inner realities rooted in the external world which make sense to them and are translated into some new external reality. My definition of a symbol can be outlined as a simple sequence of experiences: (1) I perceive external reality but in so doing I transform it, distort it, change it; (2) I try to give meaning to my perception of reality; (3) I represent that meaning in some external way, e.g., a word, a color, a gesture, an object.

These symbols, many of which are culturally inherited and never questioned by the individual, form part of the person's cognitions—the inner reality that makes sense to the individual even though that sense or meaning might be negative, destructive, or productive of unhappiness. The symbols that are an important part of our cognitions distort our experiences and our enjoyment of living. These unexamined symbols alter our perceptions and impoverish our experience of living. It seems that the current popularity of quasi-metaphysical literature such as Castaneda's (1972, 1974) books is a healthy reaction to the cultural complacency regarding our place in the world, our perception of the world, and our ability to know. To quote from *Journey to Ixtlan* by Castaneda (1972):

> "Stopping the world" [a technique taught by Don Juan in order to become enlightened] was indeed an appropriate rendition of certain states of awareness in which the reality of everyday life is altered because the flow of interpretation, which ordinarily runs uninterruptedly, has been stopped by a set of circumstances alien to that flow (p. 14).

The precondition for "stopping the world" was a total dedication to the new learning "for the purpose of pitting it against the old one, and in that way, breaking the dogmatic certainty which we all share, that the validity of our perceptions or our reality of the world is not to be questioned" (p. 14).

What cognitive therapy is all about is very closely related to this questioning of our dogmatic certainty about the validity of our perception of the world. What hypnosis does is to interrupt the uninterrupted flow of interpretation which continues to misinterpret reality for us in order to give us a chance to connect with reality in a new way. Liberated from the old ways of perceiving, we can now produce new symbols, new meanings.

Human sexuality is so complicated precisely because of the symbol-producing process involved. Unless sex therapy patients can "stop the world" regarding their previous cognitions about sex and look at it in a fresh, individualized way, all the sexual experiences of traditional sex therapy become a waste of time. The same process of symbol formation that makes us uniquely creative among the inhabitants of the planet earth also makes us uniquely miserable. We see this clearly when a person is suffering from sexual dysfunctions. But at this time in history, we have the tools to help people with these problems; we can get quickly to the inner mind where the distortions of reality, which create unnecessary suffering at the conscious level, can be modified, according to the person's mature and current existential reality.

OVERVIEW

I have placed hypnosis, especially used for sexual dysfunctions, within the general theory of cognitive therapy. This is because the latter attempts to reach the inner processes of perception, symbol formation, and beliefs affecting behavior. Hypnosis is an elegant and economical method to help people "stop the world" of reasons, analysis, logic, and excuses, and enter into a world of experiencing, inner savoring, and tasting.

The literature of cognitive therapy tends to make a distinction, at least academic, between *cognitions and imagery*. Lazarus (1976) lists both as distinct modalities. As this chapter has shown, I tend to include one in the other because more and more evidence (see Sheikh and Shaffer, 1979) points to the fact that all our "thinking" includes some form of imagery and that all our beliefs are connected with mental imagery. So, when in the previous pages I refer to cognitions, including mental imagery, I am simply trying to emphasize that an effective cognitive therapy cannot be simply cognitive, if by this we mean rational, logical, and analytical; it must also be experiential. This is the whole point of the covert techniques mentioned earlier; that is, to stop the purely cognitive functions the person is familiar with and to engage him/her in new inner experiences which will produce new attitudes leading to new behaviors.

As we have seen, cognitive therapists use mental imagery liberally but, because of the prevalent misconceptions about traditional hypnosis, they don't recognize their work as hypnotic. An example of this confusion was brought to my attention recently by Walen (1981). She wrote:

> The main difference, I believe, between the hypnotic approach and that of the cognitive therapist is how much generalization of learning can take place. In cognitive therapy, the central idea is to teach the patient to recognize and challenge a set of cognitive errors. Errors such as overgeneralization, personalization, black-and-white thinking, etc., can obviously operate in a variety of contexts—sexual, interpersonal, and intrapersonal. If the patient is trained in the art and science of cognitive therapy, the end product is hopefully an individual who has a set of tools to deal with succeeding problems as they arise.

As we have discussed in Chapter One, generalization does occur in clinical hypnosis. Moreover, everything that Walen states about cognitive therapy can be stated also about hypnosis. Its goal is, indeed, to provide new tools to the patient so that s/he can deal with new problems as they arise. From my experience, I have noticed that people who learn hypnosis get into a new way of viewing themselves—a more holistic way—realizing that they can use the new technique to improve many areas of their lives other than what brought them to therapy to begin with.

For instance, a 51-year-old executive who presented sexual performance anxiety with a woman he was seriously interested in, after a 30-year marriage had ended in divorce, reported several months later that he had applied the same techniques of relaxation and positive inner dialogue in two areas never mentioned during the six sex therapy sessions. These were when he had dental work done and when he had to take airplane trips. He told me that his dentist was amazed at his relaxation and his tolerance of pain. Regarding his flying, he confessed that before learning hypnosis he customarily drank up to five martinis in one flight because he was always "nervous" and uneasy about flying. Now he had only one drink and spent the rest of the flying time relaxing and enjoying mental imagery.

The point of this story is that many patients have had similar reactions, demonstrating generalization of learning from a very pragmatic point of view. Indeed, the interesting aspect of this type of generalization of learning is that it happened spontaneously without any prompting from the therapist at all. Perhaps what Walen described as "the art and science of cognitive therapy" consists in producing the very same effects which hypnosis produces; i.e., the switch of mental channels by which we move from secondary-process to primary-process thinking and in so doing learn to use our subconscious mind to influence our consciousness and our behavior.

Walen also emphasizes "the cognitive therapist's focus on 'secondary symptoms' or 'symptom stress' which sets him/her apart from many other schools of therapy." By this she means the high level of distress produced by the symptom itself. It is true that this emphasis is characteristic of cognitive therapists, but hypnosis is not and has never been identified as a school of therapy. In practice, though, many professionals using hypnosis are dealing with secondary symptoms, but not as intentionally as the cognitive therapist does.

My concept of negative self-hypnosis (NSH) is based squarely on cognitive therapy but extends the latter by stressing the hypnotic elements at work, both in establishing NSH and in the therapeutic work to overcome it. The hypnobehavioral approach combines several methods emphasizing imagery conditioning. The application of these concepts to sex therapy is not difficulty to understand, since traditional sex therapy has not rejected its relationship with behavior modification techniques. It seems universally accepted nowadays that sex therapy cannot limit itself to mere behavioral methods, ignoring the cognitive elements involved in the dysfunction to be treated. My point is that hypnosis is a very effective technique to accomplish swiftly and elegantly what sex therapy is trying to attain—an improved sexual functioning springing from new, idiosyncratic attitudes. The controversy is not about what we want to accomplish—the goals we have for our therapeutic intervention—but about these very interventions: Which are the most effective, long-lasting, and enriching to the whole personality? As is obvious, my contention is that hypnosis is the technique of choice.

In Chapter Four, I shall start the specific focus on sex therapy followed by concentration on the importance of sexual attitudes in Chapter Five. Chapter Six will then proceed to explain general applications of hypnosis in sex therapy, followed by three more chapters listing specific hypnotic techniques for sexual dysfunctions.

4

Cognitive processing in human sexuality

In human sexuality, self-suggestion and imagination are constantly at work. As in other areas of human interest—but, because of social restrictions, in sex even more so—humans are engaged in an inner process of evaluation, assessment, and analysis throughout the sexual cycle. This I call *processing*.

Mental processing, then, is obviously an important component of human sexuality. Because it pervades the entire human sexual experience—from the weak beginnings of mild desire, through passionate wanting and arousal, through foreplay and genital contact, to climax, afterglow, and afterthoughts about the experience—it is not possible to assign it a specific place in the sexual cycle, like desire has. Nevertheless, it must be considered a quasi-phase, completing the triphasic model proposed by Kaplan (1979). In other words, we could add a fourth phase called "processing," since many people, especially those with sexual problems, spend much mental energy and time "going over" their sexual experiences. This phase is where people usually produce guilt feelings, self-condemnation, and other negative reactions to the foregoing sexual experience, affecting desire and the whole future sexual cycle.

Walen (1980; see Chapter 2, section on Cognition and Sex) sees three *evaluation* points among her eight links of the sexual cycle, recognizing the intimate connection between cognition and human sexuality. This is stressed by Wilson (1978b), when he explains why cognitive behavior therapy is the most effective approach to the resolution of sexual difficulties.

Humans seem to be the only beings with the ability to reflect—to think about their thoughts, to know that they know, to be both subject and object of their awareness. The Cartesian *Cogito, ergo sum* could mean that people become what they think. But contrary to what some behavior therapists seem to imply, most cognition is *not* conscious, as Ellis' (1962) original model, centered on irrational beliefs, taught us.

NEGATIVE SELF-HYPNOSIS (NSH)

As a matter of fact, much of our cognition is *beyond* the awareness radius, producing real havoc in many areas of our conscious life. We allow negative "thoughts—both affirmations and imagery—to become part of our belief system. These subconscious negative beliefs can truly be said to be hypnotic in their power and, therefore, are dangerous because we cannot challenge them rationally. To review what was mentioned in the previous chapter, what I have described as negative self-hypnosis (Araoz, 1981a) consists basically of affirmations and imagery which are negative in nature. They, in turn, affect our mood, motivation, and behavior. Or, in the words of Bach (1977) through his Reluctant Messiah, "Argue for your limitations and, sure enough, they're yours." Any self-imposed limitation on what a person realistically could be, do, or have is the result of NSH—in sexual behavior, as well as in any other type of behavior. These limitations result from NSH and act as powerful hypnotic suggestions:

(1) They have been accepted by the inner mind (primary process) without critical evaluation or rational analysis.

(2) They activate negative imagery, often quasi-habitually.

(3) In the manner of post-hypnotic suggestions, they affect mood, motivation, and behavior, limiting the individual in such a way that s/he *cannot* break through those hypnotic limits.

As I (1981a) wrote before, a person using NSH without being aware of what s/he is doing, "is really unable to change because s/he is convinced that s/he cannot do it. Through a repetitive process (which the person comes to regard as quite natural and obvious) of giving him/herself negative affirmations and focusing on defeatist mental imagery, his/her subconscious has come to accept non-critically that, yes, this is impossible—perception has been distorted (and consequently, behavior has been influenced)" (p. 46; parentheses are added to the original text).

Therefore, this negative processing is the first dynamic to consider when doing sex therapy. What the person "thinks" about the overt symptom may affect the whole outcome of therapy, as mounting evidence seems to prove (Meichenbaum, 1978b). What is the hidden symptom? In other words, what is going on in the person's mind *about* his/her sexual difficulty? What is s/he "saying to him/herself" about the problem? And—never to be neglected—what *mental representations* come to mind, and are even fostered and encouraged, when the client "thinks" of the sexual problem? Thus, the first essential step in any form of clinical intervention for sexual improvement is to discover what the clients are saying to themselves about their sexuality and, especially, about their dissatisfaction or conscious desire to improve. For instance, "I wish I could improve, but this has been going on for so long that it might be too late," may undermine any therapeutic actions, such as behavioral prescriptions.

The question has been raised about the advisability of focusing on these negative mentations. Why not start right away with a positive regimen that will flood the mind with constructive messages and imagery? Doesn't the negative focus reinforce negativism? The justification for starting by looking for the presence of NSH lies in the fact that clients have seldom before verbalized this negative self-talk in a conscious way. Before the negativism is stopped, the clients must realize that they are engaged in it. Usually their NSH regarding their sexuality is linked to many significant aspects of their lives, current and past.

ROLE OF NSH IN SEXUAL BEHAVIOR

From clinical experience, it has long seemed that negativistic imagery and self-talk play an important part in sexual dysfunctions (Jehu, 1979; Kaplan, 1974, 1979; Lazarus, 1977; LoPiccolo, 1980; Rosen, Leiblum, and Gagnon, 1979). Looking at one of the first authors to concentrate on the components of what Masters and Johnson (1966) described as *spectatoring,* Kaplan (1974), dealing with the immediate causes of sexual dysfunctions, states: "To function well sexually, the individual must be able to abandon himself to the erotic experience. He must be able to temporarily give up control and some degree of contact with the environment" (p. 121). The alternate state of awareness, or of experiencing, which Kaplan aptly considers a prerequisite for "functioning well sexually," demands the opposite of NSH. Later she lists sexual anxiety and cognitive defenses against erotic feelings among the immediate causes of sexual dysfunction — both mentations belonging to NSH.

Consequently, to validate this clinical belief, a preliminary study was conducted (Araoz, 1980d) in 1978. One hundred former sex therapy clients seen during a five-year period (1974-1978) were asked to fill out a questionnaire. Only 65 responses were used because some were not returned or were incomplete. These 65 middle-class subjects had ranged in age, at the time of their sex therapy, from 21 to 67 years. The gender distribution was 39 men and 26 women. Of these, 59 were married or living together; six were unattached. All had been seen conjointly and, when appropriate, also individually. Diagnostically, 24 cases had had desire problems; 16 arousal difficulties; and 25 orgasmic dysfunctions.

The instrument used was a 20-item open-ended questionnaire, constructed with special care not to bias the responses in the direction of NSH. The 100 former sex therapy clients were contacted initially over the telephone, with the indication that this was "a study of the role played by imagination in sexual behavior." Typical questionnaire entries were:

- "What were your erotic thoughts during the weeks of your sex therapy? Please indicate whether these occurred at home or in the office; alone, with your partner, or with others."

- "Please write as literally as possible the words, phrases, memories, or images that came to your mind when you used to start thinking about sex."

- "Describe in detail how you saw yourself in your mind's eye when you thought of the possibility of having sex."

The responses were tabulated as either positive or negative. When a combination of negativistic images and self-talk belonged to the same person, it was classed as NSH. In this case, an examination of the individual's sexual diagnosis and his/her NSH determined whether there was an indication of a relationship between NSH and the sexual dysfunction.

The results are worth considering. NSH had been operative in 60 of 65 clients, with this diagnostic breakdown: in all 24 cases of desire problems; in all 16 of arousal problems; and in 20 out of 25 cases of the orgasmic dysfunctions. The five cases who did not provide sufficient evidence of NSH were thus classified because the combination of negative self-talk and negative imagery was not clear, though all of these five cases also provided evidence of negativism in one of these two areas. The religious distribution is interesting because NSH was found without significant difference among the four classifications; i.e., no religion (4), Jewish (21), Catholic (22), Protestant (13).

Although the limitations of this study are obvious and do not allow us to draw generalized conclusions, the results seem to confirm the important role of NSH in sexual dysfunctions and encourage further research in this area.

To summarize, then, when NSH is applied to sexuality, it must be considered as an important dynamic of the dysfunctional picture. When NSH appears after the sexual experience, it could be seen as a quasi fourth phase in the human sexuality cycle. In both cases, NSH applied to sexual behavior can be called negative processing and can be regarded as an important component of any sexual dysfunction. As I shall indicate later on, the distinction between sexual dysfunction and sexual disturbance depends entirely on processing—NSH in the sexual area. Negative processing is the hidden symptom which, when not uncovered, sabotages all therapeutic progress.

NEGATIVE PROCESSING

Dynamic imagery is not effective for just one type of sexual dysfunction. Since 1975, I have added self-hypnosis to all other forms of sex therapy, with excellent results. Clinically, it seems important to act as if processing were, indeed, a separate phase in the sexual cycle and to determine in great detail the self-evaluation the person has made of his/her sexual activity. The clinician should persist until the words used in the self-talk and the images connected with the post-sex mental activity become known. Most people with sexual dysfunctions do negative processing. And by "negative," I mean a self-evaluation that is not *mostly* positive, including the many who say to themselves, "I was okay, *but* I'm sure she was not pleased," and the like.

It should be noted that I am referring to negative processing, not to an objective evaluation, which might include the realistic assessment of some negative factors forming part of the whole sexual experience. The latter is conscious and leads to constructive correction so that next time those negative factors are avoided. For instance, the woman who, after sex, recognizes that she was harboring angry feelings because of a previous fight admits it and decides, for the next time, to resolve the fight prior to starting to make love. Or the man who recognizes that he had too much alcohol before sex makes up his mind in the future to be more careful about drinking when he intends to have sex. This kind of "processing" is objective, realistic, healthy, and constructive.

As was mentioned earlier, negative processing can be considered an ongoing course or a separate final phase in the sexual cycle. As an ongoing course, it refers to what goes on subconsciously in the person's mind in the sequence beginning with the perception of a sexual stimulus and proceeding to arousal, sexual activity, and, finally, the moment the person starts feeling "bad" about it. Processing is a continuum, starting with (1) stimulus *detection*, or awareness of a sexual situation, leading to (2) *labeling* it, going on to (3) *attribution*, or the interpretation of it, and ending in an (4) *evaluation*. Processing, if positive, may trigger desire, leading to detection, and so on in the same sequence again. These four steps constitute processing, reducing Walen's (1980) arousal cycle from eight to four steps, by unifying her perception and evaluation steps into one, i.e., processing, thus making her model even more elegant.

An example of processing may help. A man may say to himself, "She (*detection*) turns me on (*labeling*) by being seductive (*attribution*). It's no good for me to let a woman manipulate me in this way (*evaluation*)."

On the other hand, processing may be seen as the final phase in the human sexuality cycle. A woman may say to herself, "Sex is just not good anymore. Faking like this, just to please him, makes me all depressed," where the four elements of negative processing can be detected. It is easy to see that such processing may negatively affect desire and the entire subsequent sexual cycle.

The five major cognitive errors listed by Beck (1976; Beck et al., 1979)—selective abstraction, arbitrary inference, overgeneralization, personalization, and dichotomous thinking—may appear in any of the processing steps, whether processing is considered as ongoing or as a final phase. For instance, *selective abstraction* may take place at the initial level of *detection* ("I perceive her—only—as a sexual object") or at that of *labeling* (focusing exclusively on the "turn-on") or during *attribution* (interpreting her behavior as seductive) or as part of the *evaluation* step ("I deny myself any contact with her because 'to be seduced' is not good for me"). Similarly, it may happen with any of the other four of Beck's major cognitive errors. And it goes without saying that negative processing occurs rapidly and subconsciously, making it difficult to distinguish the four steps mentioned, unless one learns to pay attention to them. This may be accomplished through the method of dynamic imagery, to be explained in the following sections.

COMPREHENSIVE DIAGNOSIS

To limit the diagnosis of sexual problems to the many categories listed in texts, subdivided further into primary, secondary, and so on, without considering negative processing, is really to misdiagnose. It is encouraging to note that this mechanistic approach to diagnosis is increasingly rare nowadays. But, still, there is need for greater emphasis on ascertaining the presence of NSH and on processing as such. The common elements present in all of the diagnostic categories of sexual dysfunction are the cognitions comprised under negative *processing*. NSH robs the sexual experience (or even the thought of it) of playful spontaneity and contaminates it with anxiety.

Thus, the first question sex therapists ask themselves is, "Why is this upsetting this person?" To answer this they must look for NSH and how it is used in processing the sexual behavior. Being disturbed about a sexual difficulty is not a necessary correlate of the dysfunction, but a result of negative processing, This, rather then the dysfunction itself, becomes an obstacle to current and future sexual enjoyment, indeed, to sexual interest and desire.

Therefore, to diagnose sexual problems comprehensively, sex therapists must not only list the dysfunction but also, and even more importantly, investigate the processing of it, which comprises self-talk, images, and resulting mood, as the next section will discuss.

PRELIMINARY WORK

It is clear, then, from the above, that the first clinical step must be to make clients aware of their negative self-hypnosis—incidentally, not just in sex therapy but in other types of therapy as well. Only then are they able to do something about NSH. Three areas should be considered: self-talk, imagery, and mood. Regarding self-talk, simple questions like, "What do you say to yourself (or what comes to mind) when you think of your sexual problem?" go a long way toward effectively making the person aware of NSH.

Once the clients realize that they do get themselves involved in negative self-talk, the therapist can ask questions about imagery and visualization: "What mental pictures come to mind? How do you see yourself in your mind's eye when you say to yourself such and such?"

Finally, the therapist focuses on mood and feeling, or on the effect that NSH may have produced in the person's mood and feeling. Direct questions to that effect are very helpful, for instance: "How does your mood change with your negative self-talk and your negative visualization?"

Thus, clinically, it is advisable to go through these three preliminary steps, namely, to inquire about (1) negative self-affirmations, (2) negative imagery, (3) alteration of mood. It helps to linger on each of these steps, remembering that (1) and (2) may overlap and mix considerably.

Some clients do not come up with any negative affirmations—at first. One woman, 47, physically attractive, involved in community affairs, with many friends and extremely popular, kept saying that she

was a very positive person. Her sexual problem—inability to reach orgasm in intercourse—was just one of those unfortunate things; there
was nothing she could do about this, other than to put up with it. I asked her to relax for a few moments and then to close her eyes and get
into a sexual movie-of-the-mind, as Bry (1978) calls the self-hypnotic
process.

While she was doing this, her face showed increased tension and
what looked like sadness; her body became less relaxed; her breathing accelerated slightly. She was "feeling" less good. When I encouraged verbalization of her self-talk, statements like, "Again, the same
frustration," and "There is no hope," came up readily. I invited her to
return to the ordinary way of using her mind before discussing both
her mental images and her self-talk. It was a surprise to her to recognize that she was affecting her mood by her subconscious negative
processing, having taken for granted a low-level chronic depression
for almost 30 years. Her conscious positive self-talk was masking this
depression, which then had to be dealt with clinically.

The next clinical procedure is to ask clients to keep a record of their
negativism and of their experiences in therapeutic hypnosis for the
following seven or eight days—until the next appointment.

THERAPEUTIC HYPNOSIS

Next clients learn to exchange the negative self-talk and imagery for
positive alternatives. Several techniques may be applied.* I usually
ask clients to imagine themselves very vividly in a sexual scene in
which everything goes fine. In a cartoon-like fashion, or as if they
were a movie director, I suggest that they take time to build up the
positive sexual scene in great detail, including as many inner senses as
possible. I direct them to live this scene in their own mind by encouraging them to get into a sexual imagination. Without my having to
know all the details of their erotic mental scene, I suggest that their
body is fully aroused, joyfully alive; that every touch is pleasurable;

---

*Detailed general sex hypnotherapy techniques will be found in Chapter Six. The one de-
scribed here is a composite of several techniques listed in the last three chapters of the book.

that they are playfully aware of every sound, smell, taste; and that the good feelings about all this keep rising and growing.

An alternative approach, if they find it difficult to see *themselves* in a positive sexual experience, is to ask them to imagine their favorite "sex symbol"—usually a movie personality—during sex. As before, the erotic scene is built up thoroughly. Once they succeed with this vicarious scene, it is easier to go back to the earlier technique of positively experiencing themselves in their inner mind.

It should be stressed that patience and slowness are essential. Frequently, the therapist is in a hurry and the technique fails. Relaxing first is essential, since the mind is usually too overloaded with many stimuli. One should also remember that the first time usually takes longer, but that once the person has learned to relax, a simple cue, such as, "Next time you sit in this chair, you may allow yourself to relax as much as today, even more thoroughly and quicker," or something similar, will make subsequent induction briefer.

Once they are able to visualize themselves in a positive sexual experience, it is crucial to let them linger on all the good, positive feelings they experience. When they are experiencing these feelings, it is important to tie them to some simple physical act, such as making a fist, as a symbol of holding on to those feelings and recovering them anytime they are wanted. I may say something like, "From now on, any time you want to reexperience these good feelings, you don't have to think too much about it. Just make that fist as a symbol of your having the good feelings; you can fill yourself with these good feelings any time you wish."

In this way, I am helping them change the negative processing into a positive one. Incidentally, this work can be employed with any type of sexual dysfunction. As a form of mental rehearsal (see Chapter Six), it prepares the person to concentrate more specifically on sexual enjoyment and makes the person aware of his/her ability to start on the road to recovery. The hidden message in this approach is that therapy wil be very positive and its focus will be on natural spontaneous enjoyment, rather than on pathology.

As was indicated before, practice of this hypnotic technique is crucial. One frequent difficulty encountered by clients is establishing a definite time to practice this type of self-hypnosis daily and to persevere in it for a whole week. It seems that people suffering from sexual dysfunctions labor under two different, yet equally mythical biases. First, the medical myth: Sex therapy (more so than other therapies) is like a medical program, so, "Let the doctor cure me. I don't have to do too much." Next, the psychoanalytic myth, at the opposite end of the continuum: "If this thing is mostly psychogenic, it can't be resolved that easily. Many months should pass before I see any real results, since I must have a thorough understanding of what goes on before I can change."

Either bias might be labeled resistance. I prefer to take these assumptions as examples of negative self-hypnosis and handle them in the same way described earlier: (1) Notice the negative self-talk; (2) notice the negative imagery; (3) notice how they affect your mood and motivation. Then we proceed to "positivize" (1) and (2) and to become aware of any positive change in mood.

DYNAMIC IMAGERY

This type of self-hypnosis has been labeled "dynamic imagery" (Araoz, 1980b). This terminology is preferred to "imagery conditioning" (Kroger and Fezler, 1976), "movies of the mind" (Bry, 1978), "psychoimagination" (Shorr, 1974), "imagery therapy" (Lazarus, 1977), and other designations for two important reasons. First, the therapeutic intervention is based on the *dynamic* images previously produced by the client in a self-defeating manner. For instance, if the negative images discovered to be part of a man's NSH include a flaccid penis, the new imagery will disregard the flaccidity but focus on the erect penis, adding, for instance, "the energy of my pumping heart echoing in my penis, making it hard, harder and stronger; with every beat of my heart, my penis remains strong, hard, erect until *I* decide to break the heart-hard-on connection."

Secondly, the therapeutic imagery makes use of other psychodynamic elements as they are manifested in night dreams, daydreams, and fantasies of a nonsexual nature, incorporating any useful mental representations from those sources into the hypnotherapy.

For dynamic imagery to work effectively, three conditions must be met. (1) Negative reinforcement, namely, a complete disregard for the self-defeating images used previously by the client, helps to extinguish these images, so that constructive, positive, and enjoyable images can be built in their place. In the case just mentioned, the flaccidity of the penis is not brought up again; all the images used reinforce the possibility of a healthy, lasting erection.

(2) The images must be ego-syntonic—much as the affirmations to substitute the negative self-talk must be—without the therapist imposing his/her own images. In the previous example, it would have been a mistake to make a connection between the heart and the erect penis with a man who might have heart trouble or the fear of it. The new positive imagery has to be syntonic with the client's values, culture, sexual preferences, and personal history.

(3) Dynamic imagery should be intensely reinforced through persevering repetition by the patient at home. I believe that all hypnosis is self-hypnosis and that this is a skill people can learn, as explained in Chapters One and Three. Therefore, admonitions regarding practice must be firm and serious.

RESULTS OF DYNAMIC IMAGERY

I have conducted limited research to find out whether dymanic imagery is beneficial in sex therapy (Araoz, 1981b). A sample of 35 clients diagnosed as sexually abulic was exclusively treated in 1978-1979 by the method described in this chapter. They were distributed as follows: 28 males, 7 females; ages 23 to 55; all married and middle-class; 4 no religion, 9 Jewish, 13 Catholic, 9 Protestant. Of the small sample, 32 resolved their sexual problem in no more than five sessions without any further traditional sex therapy intervention. The other three needed either more than five sessions, the limit set for the study, or additional interventions—à la Masters and Johnson.

These encouraging results seem to warrant further inquiry in this area. Hypnosis for sexual abulia might be the type of specialized technique requested by Kaplan (1979) for the dysfunctions of sexual desire. But the evidence further suggests that, when it comes to processing, what is true of desire problems is also true of other sexual dysfunctions.

Cognitions, then—comprising both affirmations and self-talk, as

well as mental imagery, though not limited to visual representations—
are either inhibitory or facilitating and arousing. By identifying the inhibitory cognitions, the clinician is able to help the client replace them
with sexually facilitating cognitions. What creates the problem is not
necessarily the sexual *dysfunction*, but the cognitions that make that
problem become a *disturbance*, to follow Ellis' (1976) convenient distinction. Not all sexual dysfunctions produce sexual disturbance; the
difference lies in processing. Any sexual dysfunction, no matter how
slight, becomes problematic when evaluated as awful or catastrophic,
as Ellis is fond of saying. Even a change in sexual behavior, though
not dysfunctional, may produce sexual disturbance.

One case that comes to mind is a couple in their late twenties who
believed good sex meant reaching simultaneous orgasm. During the
first 20 months of the relationship, this had become their pattern. Being sexually uninhibited and free, they copulated every day. He had
been married before and had had many negative sexual experiences
with his former wife. Now, finally, he had found the woman with whom
he could have "good sex." But then, coincidental with his turning 30
years of age, she started reaching orgasm either before or after him,
and sometimes she didn't even reach a climax. He processed this as
"bad sex" and became quite upset, requesting psychotherapy in
order to overcome his sexual *disturbance*. This alteration in their sexual functioning—certainly not a dysfunction—was processed negatively by the man, at which point it became a disturbance.

On the other hand, there are many individuals with obvious sexual
dysfunctions (especially in problems of desire) who do not see anything wrong with them. The only reason they find themselves in therapy is the insistence and complaints of a frustrated mate, as I have reported elsewhere (Araoz, 1980a).

COGNITIVE THERAPY, HYPNOSIS, AND SEXUAL PROCESSING

Meichenbaum (1978a) has taken Coué to task because of the
latter's supposedly oversimplistic approach of "mere persuasion and
reasoning," and cited his own experiment with children who were
taught psychological mottos and ended up repeating them senseless-
ly. Unfortunately, Meichenbaum disregarded Coué's complete

treatment procedure and particularly the prerequisite of hypnosis, without which any "psychological litany" is, indeed, meaningless. Through hypnosis—when critical/logical thinking is minimized, while experiential thinking is maximized—the client's self-suggestions become much more than mere words. They become triggers for active imagining, mental rehearsal, and covert experiencing of what the words suggest. On the other hand, Meichenbaum was absolutely correct in pointing to the more sophisticated procedures developed by cognitive behavior therapy to teach people "to become better problem solvers under stress."

My intention throughout is not to contrast hypnosis to cognitive therapy or to claim superiority for the former. On the contrary, I have tried to make a case for enriching both by their mutuality. The cognitive elements affecting sexual behavior are mostly non-rational and may be reached and changed through hypnosis, combining with it some of the proven cognitive behavioral therapy techniques, such as self-instructional training, dismantling, meta-cognitive skills, and others (Meichenbaum, 1978b), which rely heavily on covert methods such as positive imagination and self-statements—in themselves hypnotic procedures, in my view. My contention is that hypnosis can and does enrich sex therapy and any specific techniques, especially cognitive behavioral ones, used as part of it, and that to ignore the "alternate state" in which many of these techniques become more effective does not make sense. There is no reason to exclude hypnosis from the interactional model of change which Bandura (1977) has called the "principle of reciprocal determinism." What is happening is that the word hypnosis seems to get in the way. Cognitive behavior therapists are, indeed, using hypnosis in most of their imagination and covert interventions, but often do not consider them hypnosis. The persistent picture of Svengali still influences the professional misunderstanding of hypnosis, overshadowing the important shifts which have occurred in the last decade or so. What Hull (1933) stated half a century ago is still true: "No science has been so slow as hypnosis in shaking off the evil association (with magic and superstition) of its origin."

Consequently, in addressing the issue of sexual processing, cognitive behavior therapy procedures will be of impressive efficacy; however, if the hypnotic aspect is underscored, these procedures will be even more effective. The historical and theoretical aspects of hypnosis (see Chapters One, Two and Three) give us enough evidence for its therapeutic usefulness and show that hypnoclinicians have been using cognitive behavioral modification techniques for many years (without labeling them so). Only recently have these been scientifically systematized.

In conclusion, the phenomenon of processing is of crucial importance in sex therapy. More philosophical questions concern the origin of negative processing: How does it start and develop? Why are some people negative in their processing, while others are not? Exploring these issues would take me too far off the main concern of this book. Suffice it to point out that a long list of serious researchers, among them Dubois (1905), Korzybski (1933), Bateson (1972), and Watzlawick (1978), have investigated the connection between inner and outer communication, between thoughts and conduct, attributing negative processing to facts of individual history, culture, and learning. Rather than thoughts and behaviors being influenced causally by interpersonal instructions, it seems that the opposite is true, namely, that elusive elements in a person's history, culture, and learning skills predispose one to the acceptance or non-acceptance of interpersonal instructions. All suggestions that are put into effect have been first self-suggestions. Or, even more precisely, only those suggestions that find an echo in the individual because of the person's idiosyncratic history, culture, and learning ability become self-suggestions and translate themselves into action.

Negative sexual processing does not *necessarily* occur because of early, unhappy sexual experiences or because of derogatory comments made by a dissatisfied partner. The therapist's task is to help a person change. To find out why the person is engaged in unsatisfying behavior is less important than to give the person the skills needed to be a better problem solver in his/her life. Sex therapy has become a particular form of behavior therapy and, as such, is an educational process in the broadest sense, providing the client with new options in learning. The focus is on the inadequate behaviors with which people are unhappy and on new ways to change them. Understanding, insight, and inner realization are merely by-products in this approach, not focal goals to attain. As it turns out, however, those by-products are often forthcoming. The point to remember is that insight *per se* does not produce change, nor *vice versa*, but that healthy change does often take place without insight, as the growing evidence provided by the behavioral modification literature continues to show (Fishman and Lubetkin, 1980).

In the next chapter, I will delve more into the issues underlying processing, i.e., sexual attitudes and values, as they have developed in our so-called Judeo-Christian culture.

5

Sexual attitudes

All sex therapists should have an awareness of their own sexual attitudes. For the sex therapist using hypnosis, this is especially important, because of the deeper interaction taking place in hypnosis. Regarding attitudes, and as an example of what I mean, one of the common characteristics of many sex therapy manuals and books on human sexuality is extreme seriousness—almost a solemn tone. This misses important aspects of the sexual experience, for instance, that of play—what I have called *sexus ludus* (Araoz, 1975, 1981c).

The need for sex therapists to be aware of their sexual attitudes, to refine them and to embrace the whole of human sexuality is imperative, simply because our clients bring to us many different sexual values. Thus, homosexuality, group sex, extramarital sexual encounters, many unconventional forms of sexual stimulation, and sexual abstinence, among other variations, may produce negative reactions in us which, though never directly expressed, convey to the client a message of disapproval and condemnation or, at the least, one of discomfort. Because in hypnosis the therapist's subconscious is engaged, perhaps as much as that of the client (Diamond, 1980; Havens, 1981), sex hypnotherapists must be especially concerned with their own sexual attitudes.

A HISTORICAL VIEW

Unless a special effort is made, humans are characteristically myopic in cultural matters: We believe that what we are familiar with is all there is, in sexuality as well as in other areas of living. Thus, frequently one hears as an explanation of the development of sexual attitudes that they have moved from procreational to affectional to recreational sex, which is generally true if one's investigation is limited to what happened in the Western world from the fourth century A.D. to the present. But a more comprehensive perspective (see Tannahill, 1980, and De Ropp, 1969) would start as far back as Neolithic times, where one finds the first evidence of sexual attitudes with the worship of the phallus as the symbol of creation, life, and cosmic energy. This practice lasted well into the Christian eras, as indicated by archeological evidence in Alexandria, from the time of Ptolemy Philadelphus (Taylor, 1954). Some even think that the crucifix was introduced as a reactionary modification of the phallic symbol. We must understand that phallic worship, and the less popular female sex worship (of which the horseshoe—a disguised vulva—is a remnant) are manifestations of very different attitudes than those prevalent in our Judeo-Christian cultures.

Playfulness is one of the aspects of sex very rarely considered in the Judeo-Christian culture. However, in sex therapy it must be stressed since the cognitive focus of the client must shift from performance to enjoyment. One common feature found in those seeking sexual therapy is their viewing sex as a worrisome problem, a source of preoccupation, limiting their perspective. They become obsessively serious about sex. Their not having fun with sex is a corollary of their problems. But spontaneous and healthy sexual desire and attraction are always pleasure-oriented and fun-seeking.

Although the biophysiological purpose of sexual attraction is, ultimately, procreation, the individual experiences the sexual attraction as an unconditioned dynamic towards pleasure and play. Developmentally, we see it in infants and children who spontaneously play with their own and each other's bodies. We observe it also in non-technological cultures, like the Chewa of Africa, the Ifugao of the Philippines, or the Lepcha of India (Beach and Ford, 1951): Among

these people, sex is primarily a pleasurable, playful activity, the bio-
logical outcome of which (children) is gladly accepted and entrusted
to the care of established and older family groups.

If toys are for amusement and play, it can be said that the most
available, permanent, and sophisticated toy for humans is their body.
This view, never emphasized in Judeo-Christian thinking, is found
again and again in the history of other cultures: in Roman Britain, in
classical Greece, among the Devadasis of the Indian sun temples, in
Tibet, in the temples of Nepal or Sikkim (Beach, 1965). In pointing
this out, I do not mean to imply that the sexual attitude of those cultures was a paragon of wholeness and health, while the Judeo-Christian is not. Historical naivete is not history. We know of the excesses
of the Greek Dionysus Zagreus celebrations or the Roman Bacchan-
alia, where abuse, violence, torture, and death were often present
(Kiefer, 1932; Licht, 1932). At the other extreme, we also know of
the desexualization process of some forms of Buddhism (Bernard,
1950; Eliade, 1958).

What I am stressing are *the differences* between what our Judeo-
Christian culture considers a normal sexual attitude and what other
human groups have believed and practiced. Sex therapists must recog-.
nize that human sexual behavior is much richer and more varied than
what they have learned. An auspicious trend is manifested by such
authors as Kassorla (1980) and Zilbergeld (1978), who dare to challenge commonly accepted notions on sexual functioning and enjoyment. An example of such notions is that of a flaccid penis not belonging in the picture of sexual excitement. The soft penis can provide a
different mode of sexual enjoyment, often ignored by the insistence
on erection. A humble attitude, based on transcultural history, will
make us discover new dimensions in sex, new joys in sex—for ourselves and for our clients.

SENSUALITY

Sex therapists have emphasized the need to awaken all the senses,
as a required preliminary for enjoyable sex. Before the person can become sexually fulfilled, his/her senses must be attuned to allow for
their healthy response to stimuli.

For instance, Montagu (1978) has commented on a problem—

non-sexual physical closeness—most males have in the Anglo-Saxon culture due to the lack of tender touching as children, which may explain "the frantic preoccupation with sex [as] a search for the satisfaction of the need for contact" (p. 192). The problem is simply that most men are uncomfortable with physical tenderness given to them, unable to enjoy mere touching and hugging, and eager "to get going" with "real" sex, namely copulation. This lack of ease with sensuality affects the woman as well, when she finds herself unable to provide tender touching because of the man's uneasiness and discomfort with it. This, often, leads her to believe there is something amiss or immature in nonsexual physical tenderness between two people who want each other sexually.

Part of shifting the attention from performance to enjoyment in sex therapy consists in teaching people to be sensual. Before sexual functioning can be healthy, people must be at ease with their physical selves and all the sensations of their bodies. It is obvious that the sensate focus, among other things, is an attempt to "sensualize" the couple with sexual problems. The sex therapist using hypnosis will start the mental sensate focus right at the office, encouraging clients to visualize sensual situations and experience mentally the comfort and joy they produce. The sooner those with sexual problems awaken their capacity to enjoy all their senses, especially touch in nonsexual situations, the easier becomes the shift from sexual "performance" to enjoyment and pleasure. The joy of sex cannot be experienced without the enjoyment of the senses. Asceticism is antagonistic to sensuality.

The playful dimension of sexual interaction is basically related to sensuality—so much so that a person not sensually awakened cannot enjoy sex as play. In sex hypnotherapy, then, after becoming comfortable with general sensual scenes, the client must be helped to mentally experience more intimate sensual (i.e., erotic) situations where the focus is on spontaneity and playfulness, on awareness of the pleasurable sensations of touching and being touched, rather than on sexual arousal. The sex hypnotherapist guides clients through these mental scenes until they are completely comfortable with them. Emphasis on practice at home is essential. And, obviously, behavioral injunctions to put into effect what they experience mentally should never be neglected both subconsciously—as post-hypnotic suggestions—and consciously.

Chapter Six will explain this in more detail. For the time being, let us return to the sex hypnotherapist's own sexual attitudes.

When it comes to sexual attitudes, we are ethically obligated to keep ourselves sexually tuned up. By attitudes I mean perceptions as they are shaped by beliefs and expectation, leading to some action. In order to take the pulse of our own sexual attitudes, it would not be beneath our professionalism to take the questionnaires proposed, for instance, by Raley (1976), for the general public. This can be quite an eye-opener for professionals. In my workshops for professionals I have used Raley's sexual attitude survey and encouraged sex therapists to discuss not only the content, but also, especially, their own feelings. Many of the workshop participants, some with many years of experience in practicing therapy, are amazed at the negative feelings they sense in themselves: reservations, reproach, annoyance, irritation, embarrassment, and so on. And often these are the same people who previously had considered themselves sexually liberated. We find that we, as experts, are not that different from our clients.

The sex hypnotherapist would do well in using self-hypnosis to improve his/her sexual attitudes. In a relaxed state, one visualizes sexual situations that ordinarily produce some tension and discomfort until the stress is gone. Then one gives him/herself the suggestion: "This is also okay; this can also be pleasurable and enjoyable. I can reject this now, but because I don't like it, not because it's wrong." In no way am I proposing that one should indiscriminately *engage* in all possible sexual behaviors. What I am stressing is that, as a sex therapist, one must feel comfortable with any and all sexual activity or lack of it which is not physically harmful for the people involved and which is engaged in voluntarily. Imagination, through self-hypnosis, gives us the opportunity to do this.

Few authors have listed systematically the myths which interfere with healthy sexual functioning, as Zilbergeld (1978) has done, but most (both popular and scientific) writers refer rather explicitly to the false and defeatist sexual beliefs prevalent in our society. Traditional sex therapists have, unwittingly, prolonged some of these myths (like the overconcern about perfect sex). There is no need to go over a whole list of these myths, since Zilbergeld, Kassorla (1980) and Bogen (1981), to cite some of the best, have done this already. I am especially interested in three basic or all-encompassing myths, shared especially by professional sex therapists.

Individual Sexual Problems

The first myth is that sexual problems are an individual matter. For instance, both Barbach (1980) and Zilbergeld (1978) conduct groups for one gender only, while Kaplan (1974, 1979) at times still exhibits a typical psychoanalytic posture, looking for the identified patient and often allying herself with "the healthy member" of the dyad. Many of the hypnoclinicians who have dealt with sexual problems (Chapter Two) have seen the spouse or the couple only rarely.

As I shall indicate in the next chapter, the cooperation of an interested partner, whether by marriage or not, in most cases facilitates the information processing and helps the couple redefine the problem as a systemic interaction, rather than as one person's fault. Even in the case where the nonsymptomatic partner is most understanding, patient and cooperative, the dynamic interaction of what takes place between the two people who share the problem must be considered, since the "goodness" of one may reinforce the problem of the other.

In one case, the wife complained about her "frigidity." She had had this condition for six years, since her mastectomy and subsequent plastic surgery at the age of 29. Her husband was so understanding that he never approached her sexually. If she was not completely into the sexual experience, he would excuse her and state that he understood. When he was invited to participate in the wife's therapy, it became obvious that this was a case of marital, not sex, therapy, the husband never having processed his feelings about her mastectomy and what he called "her artificial breast." The wife's sexual unresponsiveness only made sense within the context of the relationship (seeing the sexual symptom as a system problem).

Therapists can avoid falling into the trap of treating "individual" sexual problems by considering *most* sexual problems to be a manifestation of a systemic dysfunction. The people involved in a sexual relationship form a system; consequently, a sexual problem cannot be resolved by focusing on just the element in the system which exhibits symptoms. Even before systems theory had become popular in the mental health field, Masters and Johnson (1966) based most of their approach on systemic functioning as, for example, their process of sensate focus shows, involving the two partners in an alternate form of intimacy and closeness. More on the systemic view in sex therapy will be discussed in the next chapter.

Supersex

Another myth to be concerned with is that of supersex. Even professional authors (as two examples, see Kassorla, 1980, and the maxi-orgasm, and Goldberg, 1976, and fusion sex) give confusing messages, contradicting their own teaching. For instance, they state that sex, being a natural function, should come naturally, as if sexual behavior needed no learning (or *unlearning* of sexual myths for most adults), implying that there is something wrong with those who have trouble with sex. Connected with this is the obligatory frequency of sexual activity (the more the better) and the normalcy of being interested in all possible forms of sexual activity (try it, you'll like it). This is sexual dogmatism, as strict as the Puritanism it opposes, all in the name of freedom.

Second, some authors imply that sexual activity should (always?) fulfill us physically, psychologically, even spiritually (if it doesn't, we need sex therapy, of course), rather than emphasizing the total encounter of two human beings in a sharing situation, which is not always necessarily "great sex."

Third, the message often conveyed is that good sex always ends up at least in copulation, if not in mutual, simultaneous, orgasms. This presents a single model of good sex, instead of allowing people the freedom to experience the sexual encounter as a continuum from mere sensuality to multiple climaxes. Individuals should be allowed to place themselves at different points on this continuum, depending on many circumstances, including personal choice.

Only when people give up unrealistic expectations about sex do they become sexually free. If supersex is the goal, one is performing, scoring—not enjoying. But the mechanistic myth prevails. It was bad enough that men believed in it; nowadays more and more women are sharing the old male myth that supersex is good sex (Wolfe, 1981). Frequently, clients request help based on this mythical expectation. In those cases, it is necessary to instruct and educate clients before starting any therapeutic procedure, since the supersex myth militates against the concept of *human* sexuality, as I shall discuss in the section on intimacy. However even before educating clients, we must examine our *own* sexual attitudes, as was mentioned before.

Myths Are No More

The third all-encompassing sexual myth is that there are no longer myths about sex because we are sexually liberated. This is an especially insidious trap for the professional, leading to close-mindedness and dogmatism.

We find sex therapists who sincerely believe everybody *should* engage in sex as much as possible, with as many partners as possible. Unfair and unscientific assumptions about people's values, disregarding individual differences and choices, take away freedom in the name of sexual liberation. As Zilbergeld (1978) put it succinctly, we are missing the "sense of perspective on the role of sex in the lives of human beings. . . . In our intentness to make sex better, we forget that sex is only a small part of life . . . that in human events there are no right ways, no external scripts that will make us happy" (pp. 66-67). As he states, we need to let go of the old sexual scripts and create new ones, relevant to ourselves, that reflect our values and whole personality. Chapter Six of Zilbergeld's (1978) book on the personal conditions for good sex is a classic, which both male and female sex therapists should read.

The myth of "no myth" is dangerous at a time when ethical and moral principles are being questioned in a society which views philosophy as mere intellectual luxury, or uses it as an anachronistic way of designating non-medical doctors. Without philosophy it is much easier to accept behavioral fashions, external scripts and myths, not realizing the error. What all of us can do is, at least, question our assumptions about sex and sex therapy so that we can keep an open mind to new learning in the area about which we believe we know everything.

Connected with the three all-encompassing sexual myths mentioned is the concept of intimacy: the experience of being known as we know ourselves, of needing another, of being unconditionally accepted, of someone believing in us—all this with mutuality of feeling, communication, risk, and joy. In this respect, it is helpful to distinguish sexual behavior as being either *committed, casual, mechanical,* or *solitary,* although in each category, especially in the first two, degrees can be found. Committed and casual sex imply different levels of feeling, caring, and responsibiltiy for the other person. Mechanical sex presupposes the absence of those qualities, and solitary sex describes all forms of self-pleasuring or masturbation (as it is still called despite its negative etymology and connotations). Mechanical sex denies intimacy, though outwardly it may look like intimacy, and often becomes the main defense against intimacy.

There can be intimacy without sex, but if there is sex in intimacy, that sex is most of the time committed. All humans need intimacy, though from childhood we have built defenses against it, because intimacy makes us dependent and vulnerable. To protect us from the hurt of rejection or disappointment, we build up defensive and self-protective behaviors: denying our need, fighting to avoid closeness, refusing to take the risks of being open and close, etc. But to enjoy intimacy we must stop using these defenses. Intimacy is always difficult: It requires a commitment "in sickness and in health, for richer or for poorer" in a hedonistic society which believes in everybody's right to be happy and satisfied all the time and to have and experience everything possible. Fritz Perls' (1969) famous "Gestalt Prayer" (I do my thing and you do your thing . . .) is a good example of the popular denial of intimacy. If I don't have to live up to anybody's expectations except my own, I cannot be intimate with anybody. It would be comical to apply that "prayer" to two people sharing a sexual experience.

Intimacy means a commitment to someone else, a commitment to know the other person, to share one's inner life and one's living, including the boring and painful aspects of living. But that commitment has its ups and downs, its backs and forths. Intimacy requires work and perseverance, in spite of the "backs" and the "downs." That is why I wrote above that in intimacy sex is *most of the time* committed. There are times when it is not. The difference is that some people purposely deny feelings and intimacy in sex. Their sexual behavior is mechanized and used as an intimacy bypass. But in those who are working at intimacy, sex can be mechanical at times, although they do not make a point to avoid emotional closeness and feelings.

Ideally, then, committed sex is "the best," when the couple share much more than their bodies, namely, when the sexual sharing is a reflection of a deeper and larger communion—becoming one. Any objection to the last sentence echoes the myths and magical thinking about sex. Sex has special meaning for humans only because one perceives and welcomes the other as a human being and because of the emotional involvement.

As for casual sex, the people involved have friendly feelings for each other but they limit the exchange to the sexual experience, with courtesy, sensitivity, liking in many cases, but without further involvement or responsibility.

The topic of intimacy is important when dealing with human sexuality because sexual dysfunction can be the result of the denial of intimacy, especially for the male. When the man is engaged in mechanical sex, performance is paramount for him, and when this malfunctions the whole system breaks down and the man may be headed for a serious depression. In my experience, many men who engage habitually in impersonal, mechanical sex sooner or later start missing the qualities of intimacy: They want to feel *more*, psychologically. The sex hypnotherapist should, therefore, be vigilant about the quality of intimacy in his/her clients, even in those who are in stable relationships, since intimacy cannot be assumed. This, incidentally, is another reason to see the sexual partner with the client whenever possible.

Most sexually healthy people seem to enjoy one type of sex (either committed or casual), with occasional excursions into the other categories, namely, mechanical and solitary. But there is usually a definite mode. The therapist must discover the idiosyncratic mode of the client and hypnotically present the possibility of other types of sex by the process of mental rehearsal, to be discussed in the next chapter.

All the above does not deny the fact that some people find intimacy via sublimation and substitution in things like work, children, involvement in philanthropic, religious or civic activities, and so on. For these persons, sex may never be committed (their commitment is in non-sexual areas), but their sexual encounters are mostly casual and occasionally mechanical, or *vice versa*. As sex therapists, we have no right to doubt their declarations of satisfaction with this state of affairs. People can be—and are—happy with sublimated intimacy, especially when their sexual encounters are not purely mechanical but occasionally casual.

SELF-HYPNOSIS AND SEXUAL ATTITUDES

The main purpose of this chapter is to focus attention on the therapist's sexual attitudes. To this end the sex hypnotherapist is advised to spend some time using self-hypnosis to explore and broaden his/her sexual attitudes. The goal is to feel comfortable with any sexual difference and variety without condemning or approving it, since, in sex, good is what the people involved find so, with freedom of choice.

Only when the sex therapist is comfortable with different sexual attitudes can clients be helped, through hypnosis, to enrich their sexual attitudes and to explore their real need for intimacy or for a different type of sex. By using some of the techniques explained in the next chapter, the sex therapist helps clients to expand their perception and to become more aware of themselves with regard to their sexuality. As I shall discuss in the last chapter of the book, the problems of desire and processing are mostly problems of negative self-hypnosis, namely, of perception distorted and colored by myths, erroneous beliefs, and unreasonable expectations, leading the person to act in a way consistent with those perceptions. Our task as sex hypnotherapists is to help people be freer to choose from among a larger number of options, so they don't *have to* continue under the influence of their early programming. For this purpose, some of the exploratory techniques described in the following chapter, together with mental rehearsal, are extremely useful.

A brief clinical vignette may illustrate this point. A slim 55-year-old widow was very distressed because she had evidence that her middle son (26 and still living at home) was homosexual. By the time she saw me she had spent over two months, as she said, "unable to sleep, without appetite. . . . I lost 25 pounds." She had also stopped seeing her lover of three years and had had no sexual activity whatsoever during this time.

She was surprised that all the negative messages about sex she had received as a child and which she had successfully overcome during two years of courtship and 26 years of marriage were "in full force again." Less than two years after her husband's sudden death, she had met her lover, with whom she had joyful sex within a wholesome relationship. Now, as she put it, she felt "dead, hatred for men in general and complete dis-interest in [her] lover." She had thought that she was accepting of homosexuality but the knowledge of her son's preference had "upset a lot of things in [her] mind."

Through the process of ego-state therapy (see next chapter), she was able to accept her son's decision and choice and to recognize the perdurable nature of all the negative messages received as a child. She was also able to put the mature self in control of her life, returning to her lover, moving in to live with him, and separating from her sons (the youngest of whom was 23 and holding a good job out of state). The entire therapy process took eight one-hour sessions.

In the next chapter I shall present some general techniques of sex hypnotherapy. In the last part of the book more specialized techniques will be offered, which will serve as examples of "how to" apply hypnosis in sex therapy.

Part II

The Applications

The next four chapters, comprising the last part of the book, will describe clinical techniques applying hypnosis for sexual dysfunctions.

Since cognitive factors producing stress and anxiety are present in the vast majority of sexually dysfunctional people, as Wilson (1978b) has shown, these techniques are proposed as an essential part of sex therapy—but as a part nevertheless. Therapy, after agreement with the clients has been reached regarding reasonable and possible goals, must provide effective means of achieving those goals. Hypnosis in sex therapy is one of the means to attain those goals. Other means and techniques must be coordinated with hypnosis. This is the reason for my using what Kroger (Kroger and Fezler, 1976; Kroger and Alle, 1981) has described as an hypnobehavioral approach. Not only are the sexual partners prescribed the home assignments of traditional sex therapy, but they are also encouraged to keep records of their exercises, to schedule self-hypnosis sessions, to use a reward system, etc.

In other words, because of the current view of The New Hypnosis, clients are asked to consider themselves involved in a *program* of sex therapy in which the main factor is their commitment to themselves. The *program* consists of practicing self-hypnosis daily, of keeping records of their progress, of stopping the negative self-hypnosis, etc. The element of responsibility to self and to the spouse or partner is discussed in depth when the therapeutic contract is established.

Perhaps because so many people still think magically of hypnosis, it is crucial to stress the comprehensive nature of this approach. Otherwise, clients may misunderstand that the clinician condones their magical thinking and agrees to practice magic.

In classifying the sexual dysfunctions, I follow to some extent Jehu's (1979) system because of its common sense and all-embracing quality. I say that I follow it to some extent, since I use it merely as a base, departing from it in several cases.

Although the following four chapters may appear to use a cookbook approach, the clinical recipes are provided with the assumption that those applying them are well trained sex therapists, willing to enrich their work with these techniques. Because I am assuming a sophisticated level of clinical expertise and wisdom, it goes without saying that these techniques are guidelines which the mature therapist should feel free to modify and change, once the general principles of sex hypnotherapy have been understood and mastered.

6

Sex hypnotherapy:
General techniques

The items discussed in this chapter apply to all forms of sex hypnotherapy, either for men or for women, whether in problems of desire, arousal, orgasm, or processing. Before specifying therapeutic techniques, however, it is imperative to understand the principles underlying sex hypnotherapy.

BASIC PRINCIPLES

Principles, here, are the truths and beliefs at the root of all sex hypnotherapy. These are, first, that people know more than they think they know and have more inner resources than they realize. Erickson emphasized that we have to learn to trust our subconscious mind. The second principle is that, even with hypnosis, change in sexual functioning is, most of the time, progressive rather than dramatic and sudden. Here a brief comment will suffice, these items having been discussed previously.

Since this book is primarily for sex therapists who are willing to enrich their work with hypnotic methods and interventions, it is important to emphasize the humanistic nature of hypnosis as a special type of communication (Field, 1979) between human beings, as opposed to the mechanistic appearance of hypnotic interventions conveyed by

105

the Traditional school of hypnosis, albeit unwillingly. Nothing unconscious becomes conscious unless it is already preconscious—with hypnosis as much as by other means, in sex therapy as much as in other forms of therapy. The three corollaries of these principles relate to resistance, sensuality, and the systemic aspects of sexual functioning.

Resistance

The *art* of hypnosis relies heavily on not providing the client with grounds for resisting. Permissiveness, invitational approaches and language, and careful observation of the client's inner representational modalities all help to avoid the building up of resistances. But even the most sensitive of therapists will encounter resistance, for which hypnosis offers definite advantages, since it bypasses the critical functions of the mind. Later in the chapter special methods to deal with resistance hypnotically will be described.

Sensuality

The natural movement from sensuality to sexuality, about which the last chapter dealt, can never be ignored. Sensuality is joyous, childlike, playful fun. Again, with hypnosis, a person is able to quickly develop a "regressed sensuality" in the service of the whole personality.

Systemic Approach

The sex hypnotherapist must not only use systemic interventions but think systemically. The literature reviewed in our historical chapter is surprising in its lack of systemic awareness. A sexual symptom in most cases involves at least another partner, or—in systemic terms—the symptom manifested by one member reflects the functioning of the whole system: it not only is an indication of an existing problem in the system but also affects the future function of the whole system. If not corrected systemically, it will never allow its parts (the people involved) to function well (see Bowen, 1978).

What this means in practical terms is that many sex therapies are unnecessarily prolonged when the symptomatic client is seen (treated) alone. Though outcome studies do not emphasize this (see Hogan,

1978, and Springer, 1981), seeing the couple as a unit, according to the Masters and Johnson model, quickly provides the therapist with important information which might be long in coming otherwise. It also allows for the establishment of a correct diagnosis in terms of the type of relationship one is dealing with, since often self-diagnosed sexual dysfunctions are, in truth, dysfunctional relationships in need of couple therapy. Consequently, although in the following sections I may refer to one client, I want to stress that the sexual partner should be involved in the hypnotic techniques as much as possible. In particular, both partners should be encouraged to practice the techniques of mental rehearsal at home as an essential part of the sex therapy regimen. The systemic approach makes for participatory therapy wherein both members assume their respective responsibility for the sexual dysfunction and cooperate in correcting it. When the sexually dysfunctional client is unattached in any way to a stable partner, the techniques should, obviously, be used with the individual client.

It goes without mentioning that I am dealing with *psychogenic* sexual dysfunctions and assume some mechanism for the preventive clearance of any possible medical complication, causative of or contributory to the sexual difficulty.

CLINICAL USES

Keeping in mind the considerations of Chapter One, I distinguish three main uses of hypnosis in sex therapy: etiological, symptomatic, and for mental rehearsal (Araoz, 1979). Under the first category, both diagnostic and exploratory uses are included. The *symptomatic* uses, in turn, refer to direct, transfer, and nondirective methods of dealing with symptoms. Finally, *mental rehearsal* means an emotive-experiential form of skill-learning and action-planning, as Sanders (1976) has done with decision-making.

USING HYPNOSIS TO EXPLORE THE ETIOLOGY OF A SEXUAL DYSFUNCTION

Hypnosis, here, becomes a means of discovering, for the client's benefit, the genesis of the sexual problem (diagnosis) or the implications of it (exploratory therapy) for the whole person and/or for the system.

DIAGNOSTIC SEX HYPNOTHERAPY TECHNIQUES

Among the many techniques, I shall mention five because of their elegance and effectiveness. But first, the general method underlying the techniques will be described. It should also be noted that all the techniques to be listed in the next section, under the exploratory modality, can be employed as diagnostic tools for the couple suffering from sexual dysfunctions.

The method behind these or any other diagnostic techniques is one of progressive uncovering: (a) to identify the problem clearly; (b) to find out if there is any consciously unknown meaning for the problem; (c_1) if there is, to discover that meaning; (c_2) if there is no hidden meaning, to check whether the conscious mind is ready to invest anything reasonable to get rid of the symptom. Diagnosis usually ends here. To explore the origin of the symptom and why it started (in the case of a "message-symptom") overlaps into the next stage of therapy proper. The five hypnotic diagnostic (D) techniques follow.

D-1 Covert Sexual Examination

While in the alternate mental state of hypnosis, the client is asked to see him/herself naked in front of a full-sized three-way mirror and to describe his/her body, evaluating every part of it. The following points deserve special attention: (a) where the client starts; (b) what areas are omitted; (c) which areas are overly described or exaggerated (e.g., "feet too big" from a person with average-sized feet); (d) where the person ends his/her review. Questions can be asked, elicited by the above four points. It is also appropriate to invite associations and connections with memories of past experiences, as well as to notice the differences or similarities in the couple.

D-2 Subconscious Wisdom

Also in hypnosis, and using the naturalistic method of Milton Erickson, the person is encouraged to trust the wisdom of the subconscious so that it may reveal to consciousness the *real* nature of the sexual problem. Choices should be offered for such revelation: a dream-like scene to start presently, crystal balls or TV screens showing different aspects of the sexual problem, somatic sensations to be perceived during hypnosis and acting as a bridge to other personal realities involved in the sexual symptom. In this technique, the involvement of the spouse or sexual partner is beneficial. To illustrate, the couple in hypnosis is asked to have an induced dream* (Sacerdote, 1967) about the sexual problem or related to it. Whoever comes up first with an induced dream takes the lead and the other spouse is invited to join and participate, to enter into the first partner's dream. The therapist encourages the mental activity of experiencing as opposed to analyzing, interpreting, and intellectualizing. Usually this technique uncovers much meaningful material. As Sacerdote put it, the experience of the dream itself becomes a therapeutic attempt, independent of other interventions.

D-3 Ideomotor Questioning

With the technique of finger movements, widely known in hypnosis (Edelstien, 1981), the person is asked questions which demand a "Yes" or "No" answer. For instance, "Is the symptom a message from the inner mind?" "Is my conscious mind ready to change the causes of the symptom?", etc. There are different opinions regarding this method. I prefer to check first which finger responds to "Yes" and which to "No" (by requesting that one finger move "by itself" to indicate "Yes" and another one to signify "No"), rather than arbitrarily assigning one finger for each meaning. There is no need to complicate the procedure with another finger for "I don't want to answer," since this message is usually conveyed by the absence of finger movement, which the therapist then interprets by saying something like, "The fingers are not moving. Does it mean that your inner mind refuses to "answer?" A "Yes" or "No" signal will follow. If the therapist proceeds

---

*Induced dreams are those spontaneous cognitions that are triggered without previous outline or blueprint by the suggestion of the hypnotherapist. It may be induced by a simple invitation such as, "In the next minute or so, a dream-like scene will spontaneously appear in your mind. Just relax and don't think of thinking. Let your inner mind offer you a meaningful dream to help you understand your problem in a vital, personal way."

with caution, the "I don't know the answer" response will not be required since no question will be asked that the inner mind cannot know.

D-4 Supermemory

As if watching old family movies or slides, the client is asked while in hypnosis to observe with great detail everything that went on in the environment, as well as in his/her perceptions and feelings, which might be related to the sexual problem. The historical and relational understanding of the symptom obtained by the means of this technique is in itself therapeutic for most clients. Although this is a rather individual technique, the spouse's presence becomes supportive and often serves to elicit more information by aiding recollection.

D-5 Future Tense

The couple is invited to visualize a double screen in the mind's eye. In it, as in a before-and-after picture, each is encouraged to see and experience him/herself now (with the sexual problem still unsolved) and in the near future (without the sexual problem) and to verbalize the perceptions and positive feelings of the "future tense" experience. The stress here lies on *experiencing* the process of positive change: what happens in it; how one's life is enriched; what is acquired, etc. This usually redefines the problem and provides information about its solution.

Although in clinical practice diagnosis is an ongoing process, opposed to psychological autopsy, and the exploratory stages of therapy constantly overlap, for didactic purposes it might be helpful to see the above as hypnodiagnostic techniques. However, these may prove to be extremely useful throughout the course of sex hypnotherapy.

EXPLORATORY SEX HYPNOTHERAPY TECHNIQUES

A comprehensive approach to sex therapy is never purely mechanistic and the possibility of ramifications from the sexual symptom to other areas of the personality is ignored only to the detriment of the final therapeutic outcome. The three major exploratory methods explained by Edelstien (1981) are worthy of careful study and practice. One, ideomotor communication, was mentioned previously. The other two, the affect bridge and ego state therapy, both taken from Watkins (1978) and closely interrelated in theory, are also effective in sex hypnotherapy. The reader is referred to both authors just mentioned, since Edelstien isolates the method used by Watkins from the latter's more detailed and theoretical explanations. The importance of these two methods (they are too flexible and broad to be described as mere techniques) is that they have applicability in any stage of sex therapy—indeed, in any stage of any psychotherapy. They are described in detail later in this chapter.

Other forms of using hypnosis for psychological exploration fall more properly under the category of techniques. They all presuppose a conviction in mental processes other than what one is conscious of. In other words, the belief in the subconscious as a benign and beneficient aspect of one's existential reality is assumed, as distinct from the rather self-destructive unconscious of other schools.

E-1 Expectations

After the couple is in hypnosis, one experiences oneself in a place which is perfectly safe and comfortable but pitch dark. Reference to the sexual problem is made while the client experiences eager anticipation: Something important, enriching will happen—a meaningful surprise, something new to learn, understand, know. Slowly, and very gradually, the light grows in the place. The client looks around, sees, feels, senses new things, while the therapist keeps talking about the wonderful excitement of learning about oneself, etc., and the other spouse joins in.

E-2 Inner Vision

Another technique to uncover and explore subconscious material is to visualize an X-ray of the mind in order to obtain a new insight of what is happening now in the client's life which makes the sexual symptom possible. Similarly, one might ask the client to visualize the mind as a very complex computer and to allow any information related to the sexual problem to appear on its screen. Shorr (1977) offers a long list of very useful techniques for the exploration of subconscious processes.

E-3 The Body Speaks

Still another hypno-exploratory technique is to request that the couple think of the sexual problem and become aware at the same time of any physical sensations anywhere in their bodies. These are usually kinesthetic, gustatory, or olfactory—though, not infrequently, auditory and visual sensations are also present. Once these sensations are clearly felt, the affect aroused by them should be fully experienced. Finally, the possible connection of these sensations and feelings with the sexual problem is sought. This is done by inquiring directly, "Let your inner mind help you understand why you felt *those* sensations and emotions when you thought of your sexual problem." If the answer is not forthcoming, the suggestion is made that the inner mind can pass on this information to the conscious mind during night dreams or at an unexpected moment during the waking activities. My records for the last six years of 876 clients show that one week later, 92 percent of them report understanding of this somatic awareness and its connection with the sexual problem. Of the remaining 8 percent, 5 percent did not understand the connection the following week, but did later, and 3 percent were "failures."

With practice and greater knowledge of hypnosis, the sex hypno-therapist will devise his/her own exploratory techniques or may stay with one of the major methods, such as that of ego state therapy (see the following Transcript). The advantages of using hypnosis for exploration of subconscious processes is the bypassing of many resistances, intellectualizations, and rational excuses, since the critical mental functions are greatly minimized during hypnosis.

TRANSCRIPT: PART OF A SEX HYPNOTHERAPY SESSION
USING EXPLORATORY TECHNIQUES

(The client was Lucie, a 28 year-old woman, married five years, who in the last year had developed anorgasmia. Medical tests were negative. The husband, John, was cooperative but unable to attend

this particular session, being out of town on a business trip. His travels had started in the last year).

T: Now that you are self-hypnotized, that part of you responsible for the symptom can come forward so I and your conscious mind can talk to it. . . . Very relaxed and comfortable now, allowing that section of your self, responsible for your sexual symptom, to appear. . . . Please let that part nod your head when it is ready to talk to us . . .

L: *(Nodding)* I'm here . . . I am . . .

T: Yes? . . . What's your name?

L: *(Still nodding)* Stub. *(very slow and quite low)*

T: Is your name "Stub"? *(L nods)* Does your nod mean "Yes," that your name is Stub?

L: Yes.

T: Hello, Stub. I'm grateful that you are willing to talk to us. . . . Stub sounds like a nickname. Is it?

L: Yes, for stubborn.

T: I see. . . . Why stubborn?

L: *(Silence)*

T: You don't want to tell us?

L: Yes . . . I won't let her enjoy sex anymore.

T: That seems obvious, but why?

L: I'm stubborn . . .

T: Yes, Stub, but I know that you have Lucie's best interest at heart. So if you won't let her enjoy sex anymore, I know there is a good reason. But I don't know the reason. Will you tell me?

NLP

L: Suspiciousness . . . *(A faint smile comes upon her face).*

T: Tell me more. I don't understand.

L: Dummy, like Lucie, eh?

T: Can you tell me what suspiciousness means?

L: She's too suspicious of John.

T: Let's understand this, Stub. You don't let Lucie enjoy sex because she's too suspicious of John. Right?

L: Yes. She just can't. Too suspicious.

T: If she stops being so suspicious, will you let Lucie enjoy sex again?

L: Yes . . . definitely, yes.

T: Stub, you are one of the many parts of Lucie who are usually hidden but who take care of Lucie and protect her. . . . Is there any other part that can help her *not* be so suspicious?

L: No, I can help. . . .

T: Can you tell us how you can help Lucie?

L: I *am* helping . . . much suspicion, no orgasm . . . (*Long silence*)

T: You don't have anything else to say, Stub? (*Silence*)

L: Stub is gone . . .

T: Too bad, I wanted to thank Stub for the help given. . . . Anything you want to say, Lucie?

L: No, I know what I must do. . . .

T: All right, then, whenever you want you may bring yourself back to the ordinary way of using your mind, to this room and hour and day. . . . By the time your eyes open, you'll feel terrific.

Lucie then explained that she had really understood now how unfounded her suspiciousness of John was. She didn't like his traveling, was mad at him because of it, and allowed all sorts of negative imagery about him to fill her mind. She knew now that she had to work systematically to control those cognitions. Three more sessions with the couple were enough to overcome the problem by means of mental rehearsal and ego-strengthening techniques.

SYMPTOMATIC USE

This refers to the more or less direct focusing on the symptomatology rather than on its subconscious implications and reasons. This is the best known use of hypnosis in medical and psychological practice, as well as in popular nonprofessional applications of the skill.

Traditional therapists are usually concerned with symptom substitution when the focus of therapy is on the alleviation or removal of a symptom. Several authors in the field of hypnosis have dealt with this issue (see Hartland, 1975; Kroger, 1977; Wolberg, 1964), pointing to the fact that the evidence is practically nonexistent for believing that the removed symptom is substituted by another one. As a matter of fact, the evidence seems to confirm what sex therapists have long known; i.e., that very often the removal of the symptom enhances the whole personality (Fishman and Lubetkin, 1980). The three symptomatic uses of hypnosis will be described, assuming that there is no clear clinical indication *not* to focus on the symptom.

DIRECT SYMPTOMATIC TECHNIQUES

The combination of imagination and suggestion is at the root of all symptomatic techniques. As was mentioned previously, all suggestions must be ego-syntonic and idiosyncratic, based on what the client has revealed initially. Thus, before working directly on a symptom, the sex therapist must know how the client thinks this change will affect his/her life, what expectations and fears the person has about the change, what advantages or disadvantages the person imagines will accrue from the removal of the symptom, and so on.

*NLP
well
formed
outcome*

P-1 Ego States

With this in mind, one can profitably use a form of ego state therapy, à la Watkins (1978), by visualizing the symptomatic self negotiating or fighting with the nonsymptomatic self, the latter overpowering the former (see preceding transcript). If the person visualizes the non-symptomatic self as weak, time should be given to the strengthening and growth of that part of the personality before engaging it in a negotiation or fight with the symptomatic self. The spouse or sexual partner is invited to share in the experience of the other. I prefer to have them work hypnotically (both hypnotized), though in several cases one spouse was not hypnotized but still participated with the other.

P-2 The Message Symptom

A variation of this technique is to suggest, once the person has entered hypnosis, that the symptom will appear in his/her mind as something concrete: a living thing (human, animal, angel, etc.), a color, a sound, a shape or form, or a combination of all these things. It is important to involve the spouse or partner in meeting the "materialization" of the symptom and in cooperating towards its change or disappearance. Depending on what appears in the person's mind, the therapist will make appropriate suggestions. In one case of prematurity, the man "saw" his problem as a small rodent quickly chewing inside of him. Asked what the rodent was chewing, he said, "Something like a line . . . an electric cable." Asked about the cable, the man reported that it connected with his penis and kept it from discharging. He was told to strengthen the cable, to see it protected by a strong metal covering. When he did not respond to this suggestion, the rodent was said to be electrocuted so that it could not damage him any longer. This was accepted and the symptom disappeared the next time he engaged in sexual intercourse. *

P-3 Wellness

Another direct technique in sex hypnotherapy is to help the individual connect mentally with all the health forces in the body. With great detail, the health and healing processes in the body (involving the immune system, the spleen, liver, kidneys, and other inner organs) are referred to symbolically: like a stream of a warm, gentle, but powerful fluid, or like a healing light, and so on. These health forces, then, are specifically channeled to the sexual organs and their connections with the nervous and muscular systems. The flow of the health forces is emphasized, healing, strengthening, rejuvenating the whole sexual apparatus from brain to genitalia. I stress the ease with which the body functions when it is healthy, the fact that sex is a normal, natural function of the body, that the person has the inner power to free the health forces to do their work in the body, that they will give the person a richer share in living, and so on. I also encourage the spouse to repeat some of the above suggestions to the partner and to make reference to his/her own health forces joining those of the partner.

As was said before, I am presenting these techniques serially for didactic reasons. In clinical practice I find myself combining several of

---

*Depending on the therapist's theoretical persuasion and the client's motivation, one may end treatment at this point (once the symptom is no longer present), or one may proceed to investigate its symbolic meaning. If the latter is the case, one of the general hypnotic techniques for psychological exploration may be used.

these, almost never using only one technique by itself. This is especially true of the direct symptomatic hypnotic interventions. Even after the symptom is removed, I invite the couple to find out what it meant, why it had appeared originally, etc. Most couples are curious and continue therapy.

TRANSFER SYMPTOMATIC TECHNIQUES

In general, this approach refers to the hypnotic production of an experience in one part of the body to be transferred to another. Thus, in medicine, one way of producing hypnotic analgesia is to obtain numbness of a hand first and then to transfer that lack of pain sensation to the affected area. In the next two chapters, hypnotic transfer techniques will be discussed for both lack of vaginal lubrication and erectile dysfunction.

T-1 Affect Bridge

Watkins' (1978) affect bridge, mentioned earlier in the section on exploratory techniques, is a good example of a transfer technique: The client is directed to experience the unpleasant feelings connected with the sexual problem, to intensify them until they become a memory bridge to a previous event in the client's life which produced the same effect. This feeling, common to both the current situation and a previous ego state, becomes the bridge to gain control over the symptom to be removed, as the transcript at the end of this section illustrates.

T-2 Relaxation

A very simple transfer technique is based on relaxation. The client is encouraged to relax (and, when necessary, guided progressively through different muscle groups, or by the method of muscle tension and release) and is encouraged to experience him/herself getting even more deeply relaxed in a comfortable, beautiful, and safe place of his/her choice, preferably outdoors, where s/he can feast all his/her senses while relaxing deeply. Feelings of wellness, confidence, inner strength, and security are encouraged both by the therapist and by the partner when available. Then, that general relaxation is focused on the sexual area, going back to the relaxing scene whenever there is some tension developing, returning to the focus on the sexual area when the tension is released. This process continues until the person has transferred the general relaxation completely to the sexual area. At this point it might be useful to mentally introduce the client's sexual partner and employ the same process for obtaining relaxation while "thinking" of a sexual encounter.

TRANSCRIPT: PART OF A SEX HYPNOTHERAPY SESSION USING TRANSFER TECHNIQUES

T: Now that you are so deeply relaxed . . . isn't it a good feeling? . . . (*Client nods*) Allow yourself to think of your sexual difficulty (*C. frowns, thinking of his erectile problem. At 32, he obtains an erection but if he does not copulate immediately, he loses it and cannot recover it for a long time. Endocrinological and urological tests are negative*). Become aware of these negative feelings (*C. has a weak, joyful smile*) . . . They make you smile? (*C. shakes head*). Would you tell me now, please what is happening?

C: Good feelings . . .

T: Think again of your sexual problem. You have good feelings when you think of it? . . . (*C. nods, smiling*) Let those good feelings, then, take you back in time, as far as you must go, to find another situation when you had . . . these feelings . . . in your past . . . Forgetting everything else for now . . . (*C. becomes serious again*)

C: Boys . . . one guy . . . not gay.

T: Tell me more, please . . . (*Silence while C. seems to relax*).

C: Feels good . . . enjoy . . . (*He sees himself at eight or nine years of age with two other naked boys. There is sexual play and erection on his part. He wants to try anal intercourse with one of them, but the third comments on the pain that would cause both of them. His penis becomes flaccid and he feels good about it. In his mind, more caressing, oral sex, and physical closeness ensue, but he has no other erection and he feels very good about it because he does not want to hurt his friend or himself.*)

T: Stay with that very good feeling now. You are forgetting all about the previous scene now, and stay just with the good feeling. All you feel is the good feeling. And let yourself go back, if you must, to another, earlier time when you felt that good feeling . . . (*C. smiles like a little boy and slightly changes posture as if he were lying down on his back.*) Tell me where you are, please . . . (*Age regressions, like this, never obliterate communication with the adult self in hypnosis*).

C: Baby . . .

T: Who is with you? . . .

C: Mommy . . .

T: What is happening? . . .

C: Change . . . good . . . (*with a broad smile*) . . . caress . . .

T: Now stay with the good feelings but forget everything else . . . just the good feeling. . . . . . Now, come back to the present, bringing the good feeling with you. . . . That good feeling will make you understand more about yourself . . . will make you happier with yourself.

When he finished the hypnosis experience, he explained that now he had learned two important things about his sexual symptom, namely, he had connected copulation with hurt, and being soft and flaccid while making love with good feelings similar to those of being changed, powdered, and caressed as a baby. With this new information, his sexual activities with his wife (who had been present at this session) began to improve. He allowed for healthy regression in sex but he also started enjoying the pleasures of mature copulation. In four weeks he was dismissed from therapy.

In this case, there was a double affect bridge, first through negative feelings, then through positive ones, leading the client to remove the symptom in an intelligent and fully human way.

NON-DIRECTIVE SYMPTOMATIC TECHNIQUES

Under this rubric I include all approaches which follow more or less closely the Ericksonian model of naturalistic hypnosis or Hartland's (1975) indirect hypnotic maneuver of ego-strengthening. The general idea is to help the individual with a sexual problem to stop focusing mental energy and attention on it and to concentrate on his/her real resources, strengths, and positive qualities. This is a way of counter- acting negative self-hypnosis and of putting the client in touch with the neglected positive side of his/her life, not by making intellectual as- sessments of pluses but by experiencing them in one's inner mind, by savoring and enjoying them. This approach is valuable in combina- tion with any of the others; however, with those preoccupied—almost obsessed—with their sexual dysfunction, the non-directive tech- niques are best. A. M. Pelletier's (1979) image of a majestic tree with which the person identifies is a good example of this approach. He takes clients through a slow sensory enjoyment of a big, mighty tree, admiring its beauty and describing all the details connected with it: rich foliage, birds singing, strong roots and so on. Then he makes the association of all the tree's virtues with the client: "*You*, like *that* tree, have been made *stronger* by the vicissitudes of life. Like the tree's branches, *you reach out* for help and *energy*. You, too, can offer *shelter* and *help* to others. Within *you* are the various *functional* sys- tems to make the *whole you stronger and healthier*. But now, *think deeply, you are more than that tree. You can think, you have mobil- ity, you can be discreet, you can make decisions, you can love and be loved, you can do so many, many things* that tree cannot do. Sense *your power, your strength, your abilities. Be grateful for you.* Think of *all you are!* Now, please, *relax deeper and deeper* as you contemplate your strength (p. 34, original emphasis)."

This approach is apt to trigger a multitude of subconscious pro- cesses in its non-directness.

It is not difficult to adapt these concepts of strength, life, healthy functioning and the like to particular sexual problems. By getting in touch with one's inner resources and vitality, one is able to establish a new subconscious connection between those inner realities and one's sexual symptom. With hypnosis, then, one can activate those hereto- fore hidden powers and direct them to the sexual symptom, bypass- ing intellectualizations and "rational" objections.

This was the case of Roger, a 43-year-old blue-collar worker who had psychogenic erectile difficulties with his second wife. Through the process of hypnotic ego-strengthening, he awakened a new positive self-esteem he had never experienced before in his life. With it, his sexual problems disappeared—which, in turn, reinforced his new self-esteem. A new "virtuous cycle" was thereby developed, giving him new motivation for personal growth and emotional enrichment. Among the immediate results of this change, Roger took steps to complete his high school education, made constructive efforts to improve his social image, and became more selective about his friends.

The non-directive use of hypnosis facilitates the freeing of positive subconscious dynamics, which soon benefit the whole person, even when the initial focus was on a particular sexual symptom.

HYPNOSIS FOR MENTAL REHEARSAL

Maltz (1960) popularized mental rehearsal and in his wake came mental sports (see Nideffer, 1976), and imagery for self-improvement (Barber, 1980)—even for making more money (Hill, 1966). In the area of sexual functioning, hypnosex (Araoz and Bleck, 1982) is basically hypnotic mental rehearsal. In a nutshell, this technique consists of the use of time progression to the set of circumstances in which the client sees him/herself thinking, interacting, and behaving in a sexually satisfying way. This Virgilian process of "seeing oneself having changed" (possunt quia posse videntur) is, in itself, ego-enhancing and self-metamorphosing. People become psychically stronger when they see themselves in their mind's eye being what they want to be (Lazarus, 1977).

Consequently, the couple (rather than merely the individual) are taught to experience themselves in the future by means of mental rehearsal, enjoying the reality of joyful sex which will be theirs. All inner senses are involved in this mental exercise, lingering on every pleasurable touch and sensation, on every enjoyable smell and taste, on every pleasant sight and feeling. The sex hypnotherapist need not become a professional voyeur, as it were, by getting into every detail of the positive sexual experience the couple is reviewing in their mind. General suggestions about every sensation, as mentioned, are sufficient.

It should be stressed that they must practice this exercise on their own, both alone and as a couple, doing it in great detail, including all circumstances surrounding the positive sexual experience, such as the place where they see themselves, the time of day, food or drinks they may be sharing, music playing, incense or perfume in the room, etc. Barber's (1980) research indicates that positive change is facilitated by this technique because the client identifies progressively with the "new" self—in this case, with the new *sexual* self. The current, problematic self becomes more and more foreign to the client; his/her mind becomes more dissociated from the current, symptomatic self.

Mental rehearsal in sex hypnotherapy should always be included, no matter which other techniques are used. When clients find it difficult to experience themselves mentally as changed, one suspects secondary gains—often subconscious—which will require approaches focusing of the etiology of the dysfunction.

NLP

RESISTANCE

A few final words should be added about the general hypnotic techniques to handle resistance. First, we should remember that any action or lack of action directed at perpetuating the symptom or situation the person complains about is resistance. Any way of continuing the self-imposed limitations to happiness, fulfillment, satisfaction, and personal growth is resistance.

Therefore, in sex hypnotherapy we encounter two basic possibilities: One, when the therapist senses *the presence* of resistance, and two, when the therapist suspects *the possibility* of resistance. For the latter case, as was mentioned earlier in the chapter, a permissive approach is facilitative: The less there is to resist, the less resistance will appear. So, the hypnotic suggestions may go something like this: "You don't know for sure in your conscious mind what your inner mind wants. Perhaps your symptom can't go away now because your inner mind is using it for something your conscious mind doesn't know," and so on.

When the therapist is, however, in the presence of resistance, two courses can be taken, either to suggest new possibilities or to explore the *subconscious* reasons for the lack of progress. An example of the former approach was given earlier (P-2) when the man did not respond to the suggestion of protecting "the electric cable" he visualized as connecting his brain to the erect penis and controlling his ejaculation. Another suggestion (that of the rodent being electrocuted) was introduced, rather than exploring possible subconscious dynamics for the rejection of the first suggestion. As a general rule in sex hypnotherapy, one should introduce a new suggestion (always prefaced by "Perhaps you could focus on . . . ")—or even several suggestions— before proceeding to a more analytical level. It is surprising to observe how often people who reject the first suggestion welcome the second or third.

In mental rehearsal, for instance, when the person cannot visualize the new asymptomatic self, it is possible to suggest a sex movie of someone who looks very much like the client. The client is watching the movie, more and more realizing how much like him/her the person in the movie really is. Often, spontaneously, the client changes the person in the movie to him/herself. This indirect approach may be used also in other techniques, such as F-1, Dynamic sexual imagery (Chapter Seven) or A-2, Revivification (Chapter Nine).

CONCLUSIONS

The general techniques for sex hypnotherapy listed in this chapter are mere possibilities. One of the rewarding aspects of using hypnosis is that one can be so creative and inventive.

My insistence on a systemic approach does not mean that individual clients should not be seen for sex therapy. In many cases, it is clinically advisable not to see the two members of the system. However, systemic *thinking* must always be the preferred choice when a client is involved in a relationship. Only in the cases of non-relational sex (either alone, in groups, or with passing and casual partners) must we focus more specifically on the individual.

Familiarity with the techniques listed in this chapter, through careful, supervised practice in the beginning, will convince the sex therapist of their great usefulness.

The final chapters of the book will present specific hypnotic techniques for differential sexual dysfunctions. The frequent appearance of these general techniques will be noted throughout the following chapters.

7

Hypnotic techniques for female sexual dysfunctions

This chapter, as well as the next one, limits itself to gender difficulties, presenting hypnotherapeutic techniques specifically designed for differential dysfunctions of women. Only the most common dysfunctions will be covered, i.e., vasocongestive dysfunction, vaginismus, preorgasmia, dyspareunia, and inadequate pleasure. The sex hypnotherapist familiar with these techniques will be able to devise new ones for less common female sexual problems, based on the ones listed here.

VASOCONGESTIVE DYSFUNCTION (VCD)

Kaplan (1974), who first distinguished between arousal problems in women and orgastic dysfunction, called it either *general sexual dysfunction (GSD)* or *female sexual unresponsiveness* (in her illustrated manual, 1975). Jehu (1979) coined the term I am using, which is more precise and focuses specifically on the arousal problems, without considering its possible roots in sexual abulia, as Kaplan's terms may imply. VCD refers to inadequate physiological arousal, namely, absent or partial genital vasocongestion with light or no lubrication,

124

leading the woman to derive little or no satisfaction or erotic pleasure from sexual stimulation. The woman wants sex, but her body does not cooperate and, as a consequence, she can't enjoy it.

Assuming that this is the correct diagnosis (negative gynecological findings, adequate sexual interest and desire, no serious relational problems or deep-seated personality deficiencies), hypnotherapy is effective. Though, as explained, this dysfunction has often been considered as part of "frigidity," implying lack of interest, inadequate arousal, and even anorgasmia, the literature offers enough of a pattern to extract from it effective sex hypnotherapy techniques, according to my earlier comments in Chapter Two.

One general and two specific techniques will be described, although in clinical practice they can be combined effectively. It goes without saying that some of these may be used for other female sexual dysfunctions as well.

F-1 Dynamic Sexual Imagery

In hypnosis, the woman first alone (although her sexual partner, if she does not object, and if at all possible, should be present from the first session on), and later together with her partner in hypnosis, is asked to mentally review her *progression* from her first thoughts of sex, through the initial steps of physical closeness and sexual desire, lingering on this. The woman may need to see herself wanted, loved, cared for by her partner, but still fully clothed. She should be helped to tarry in a mental scene where the stress is on her positive feelings ("It feels so good to be together, to hold each other; you want him so much, time stands still in his arms, his embrace, his kiss," and so on). Depending on her comfort and relaxation with this type of quasi-erotic scene, the therapist proceeds further ("You want more contact with his skin, your living body close to his, warm, comforting. It feels so natural to be partially undressed together, so good to feel the warmth of his body, skin to skin in mutual caring, enjoyment. The joy of being alive, making love," and similar statements). Constant input from the client is necessary, as well as keen observations of any physical changes possibly indicating discomfort. When the therapist is aware of a movement or facial expression which might reveal tension, s/he should ask ("Are you with it?" "Can we proceed?" "Is everything pleasant?" or other such questions).

In one case, a client was grimacing very noticeably, and I feared she was feeling uncomfortable with her hypnotic imagery. When asked, she replied: "The sweater, take off the sweater," and smiled. My fear was unfounded. Had I gone on the assumption that she was moving away from the sexual scene, I would have interrupted what was an important step in her mental sexual involvement, namely, encouraging her partner to undress her.

Finally, the therapist helps the person to focus more concretely on her body and her genitalia ("It's nice to be so relaxed and still so aroused. Yes, my body wants sex as much as my mind. I feel it inside of me, lubricated and open and warm. And it feels so good. My body is becoming more and more ready, with every breath I take, with every second that passes, open, warm, moist. It's so wonderful to feel this inner peace, this physical desire; my body open, eager, ready," etc.).

The post-hypnotic suggestions should relate this exercise to appropriate situations when she is with her sexual partner ("More and more, where sex is possible between us, my body will react in the same wonderful way. I'll feel relaxed, terrific. My body and my mind in harmony of desire, physical contact, pleasure, excitement," and so forth). All these statements, provided as mere examples, are repeated or prolonged according to the client's tempo and need. She is firmly encouraged to practice this exercise at home. Frequently, it is helpful to tape record the hypnosis part of the therapy session, so she can practice at home with greater ease. In this case, instructions should be given regarding "getting into it," not just listening to the audiotape. Also, the person should be asked to return the tape at the next session, so the therapist doesn't lose control of who uses his/her tape and how it is being used.

This is a general technique, which, with appropriate changes, can be used for other sexual difficulties, always in combination with the more specific techniques which follow. As stated earlier, the sexual partner should be invited to participate in the hypnotic sessions as soon as the client is ready. It is obvious that in such cases the therapist will accommodate the statements accordingly.

F-2 Untensing

Similar to T-2 in the previous chapter, but focusing on the pelvic area, this technique emphasizes the health forces in the body, freeing them through imagery to flow naturally and powerfully. Therefore, once the woman has entered hypnosis, the therapist may follow T-2 technique and combine it with P-3 in the same Chapter Six. The method should move gradually from a general relaxation to the relaxation of the pelvic area, taking different parts at a time ("the walls of your vagina, the depths of your vagina"). It is not necessary to use technical expressions or to be anatomically exact (unless the person knows anatomy), since the goal of this technique is to free the woman from the mental tensions that inhibit the normal functioning of her body in a sexual situation.

Again, as in F-1, it is important to give post-hypnotic suggestions related to erotic situations with her husband or sexual partner. The latter should, when possible, be present during the hypnosis sessions in order to help in the relaxation and untensing, since often his tension contributes to the woman's difficulty.

F-3 Salivation

This technique is based on the physiology of feminine sexual arousal. Normally, physical and/or psychological erotic stimulation produces a vaginal lubrication. No glands exist in the vaginal mucosa or submucosa, but a well-developed capillary system surrounds the basal membrane. During sexual stimulation these capillaries are engorged with blood, as are other genital organs. Transudation occurs and liquid appears on the vaginal wall. Though this physiological process is complex, the woman experiences it as becoming moist, a sensation resembling salivation when, thinking about a delicious food, the mouth waters. The physiology of these two phenomena is very different, but the subjective experience is not. Based on this subjective analogy, the woman in trance is helped to associate salivation with vaginal lubrication. Increased salivation is effected by suggesting in hypnosis a healthy food the woman likes. She has to become aware

of her physiological ability to produce salivation through mental imagery. Then suggestions are given, associating salivation with vaginal
lubrication: "As your mouth increases the flow of saliva, so will your
vagina next time you are feeling sexual . . . and every time you feel
sexual, your vagina will increase its moisture. It'll be a good feeling, to
be moist, to feel warm and open, moist and ready; every time you
are sexually aroused, your body will respond so wonderfully," and
so on.

This is one of the "transfer techniques" mentioned in the previous
chapter. A bit of practice may be needed to effect salivation, but the
results of this technique are positive, quick, and lasting. As mentioned
above, I involve the woman's husband or sexual partner whenever
possible and encourage them to practice this: first, as described above;
then, experiencing the vaginal lubrication but without rushing to copulate; and finally, effecting moisture of the vagina through self-hypnosis, ending in a mellow, comforting sexual encounter with intercourse.

VAGINISMUS

The involuntary spasm of the sphincter vaginae and levator ani
muscles (the outer third of the vagina and the perineum) when an object, including the erect penis, is brought in contact with the inner labia, is treated effectively with sex hypnotherapy. Except for the last
technique, the previous ones mentioned (F-1, F-2) are also beneficial
for vaginismus. Relaxation (F-2) is essential to remove fear and possible guilt from the sexual experience. The mental image of the muscles
controlling the whole pelvic area, and especially the vagina, as rubber
bands that can become untense may be helpful. However, the best
approach is to ask the woman to describe how she feels that tension. If
she says, for instance, that it feels like a tight knot, that image should
be used, and slowly she can be helped to visualize the rope or cord
with the knot loosening up until there is no knot.

Also for vaginismus, the exploratory techniques mentioned in the
last chapter (E-1, E-2, E-3) are often beneficial. Many clients remark
that they don't understand what's wrong with them or what's happening in their body. ("I have no control over it," "I don't know where it

comes from," are typical comments.) Such comments are a cue to the sex hypnotherapist to help them explore what's taking place.

The summary of a clinical case may elucidate this approach. After three years of unconsummated marriage, Ann, 25, had had several forms of treatment, over a period of five years, including vaginal dilation, medication, psychoanalytical psychotherapy, and behavior modification—all without success. Since Ann arrived with quite a pessimistic outlook, a combination of several etiological techniques was used; these included, among others, subconscious wisdom with ideomotor questioning (D-2 and D-3), future tense (D-5), and mental rehearsal, and especially, ego state therapy. Ann reacted very well to the latter but some of her "inner parts" responded only ideomotorically, and others refused "to talk" to me but insisted on doing so with her husband. As homework assignments, relaxation exercises were prescribed, focusing on the future, when copulation would be desired and enjoyed. Ann practiced faithfully and her husband cooperated very well.

Past material, difficult to corroborate because her aunt, who had raised her, was dead, emerged in the second of eight sessions. This had not come up before in her previous therapy. Ann relived a scene in which someone (her aunt?) hurt her at the age of five or six by inserting two fingers in her vagina in the process of bathing her thoroughly. (Consciously, Ann did remember her aunt as being obsessive about body cleanliness.) This had started her vaginismus.

As a clinical observation, it is to be noted that material like the above, obtained through hypnosis, may not be historically accurate but is relevant, nevertheless, because it comes from the person who is suffering the distress for which therapy is sought.

In another variation of ego state therapy, Ann as the mature woman encountered the little seven- or eight-year-old girl. Then, in a hypnotic age succession, she reviewed different times in her life—at ages 12, 15, 17, 18—when during self-pleasuring, petting, or early attempted intercourse her vagina had reacted spasmodically in a conditioned response. The mature Ann was always there, in her recollection exercise, to advise and help the younger Ann. With her current understanding and resources, she was able to help the adolescent self in her inner mind.

After the third session, she reported that she had been able to insert her fingers in her vagina without any problem several times—a practice which had always been filled with anxiety when she had tried it before as part of one of her previous therapies. She also had inserted a tampon for the first time in her life.

The progress continued: Perfect relaxation with manual stimulation by the husband was reported in the fifth session; brief insertion of the penis was reported in the sixth session; and total copulation was reported in the seventh session. Two follow-up phone calls were made one month and four months after the eighth session. The gains were maintained. Through referrals made by Ann, she kept confirming her gains for five years after her therapy, when she moved out of town.

PREORGASMIA (DYSORGASMIA)

When the woman is interested in sex and desires to enjoy it, is erotically stimulated and aroused, but cannot reach climax, she is said to be preorgasmic. The choice of this description gives the woman a sense of hope: She still has not attained orgasm, but she's just short of doing it, and can learn to enjoy the climactic experience.

As in all the other dysfunctions, it is common to find this problem in combination with one or more sexual difficulties, raising questions as to cause and effect. On the other hand, what is to be kept in mind is that lack of orgasm doesn't necessarily mean lack of sexual enjoyment, as Butler (1976) found in the 195 women she studied: 73 percent didn't always need orgasm to enjoy the sexual contact; 39 percent obtained relief of sexual tension even without climaxing.

Hypnotically, the techniques described previously are also effective in orgastic dysfunctions. Here I want to discuss a specific technique for this condition.

F-4 Body Trip

This technique consists in imagining, while in hypnosis, a trip through the genital areas. The hypnotized woman is asked to see herself inside her vagina, as if she were, for instance, a building inspector checking every detail of this beautiful chamber or tunnel or corridor, starting from its entrance. She is to see herself feeling its entrance, roof, and walls, tapping its sides and end, checking any special points (purposely leaving it up to the client to make sense of the phrase "special points" while thinking of her genitalia). The woman is encouraged to check which areas or points respond with "nice sensations." Is there any pleasure anywhere? Which areas respond with pleasure to touch, to tapping, to rubbing, to pressure, and to any other form of contact?

All along, the sex hypnotherapist must get input and feedback from the client, so she can be paced properly and is not rushed. Simple questions like "Are you focusing on this?" or "Are you still with it?" provide the clinician with the necessary information on how to proceed. When she "discovers" where pleasure is generated, she is encouraged to visualize pleasure as "a thing" (a sound, a sensation, a perfume, a color, a taste, or a combination of these sensations), to linger on it, to get into it, and to increase it or diminish it a few times.

When she is comfortable with this mental experience of pleasure, and still relaxing in hypnosis, her lover or husband is introduced in the mental imagery. Then her sexual partner becomes associated with pleasure, either first by his touching (depending on the woman's form of orgastic dysfunction) or directly by his genital contact. This mental scene is prolonged until the client is relaxed, comfortable, and happy with the experience. She is encouraged to repeat this self-hypnosis exercise as often as possible and, when feasible, together with her husband or sexual partner.

The post-hypnotic suggestions should be related to the actual situation of copulating and enjoying it. Even at the risk of being repetitious, it must be said that the efficacy of this technique depends on a correct diagnosis. If the dysorgasmia is a manifestation of relational conflicts, these must be addressed first, before the sexual problem is treated.

DYSPAREUNIA

Although in most cases some organic pathology causes pain during and after coitus (either in the labia, the clitoris, the vagina, or the internal pelvic organs), psychological factors often contribute to the dysfunction. Therefore, in conjunction with medical attention and in co-operation with the gynecologist, the nonmedical sex hypnotherapist will find the relaxing techniques (F-2, F-4, and T-2) especially helpful. However, in cases where the gynecological findings are negative, one should carefully evaluate the sexual (total) relationship with the partner, on the one hand (using some of the exploratory techniques) or, on the other hand, the general personality of the woman. Some studies (Winokur and Leonard, 1963) correlate certain types of conversion disorders with dyspareunia. Finally, the therapist must consider the possibility of a conditioned response, which is a good example of negative self-hypnosis: The expectation of pain because of some pain experienced in the past, though the organic cause is no longer present, produces pain once more. In this case, the method to counteract negative self-hypnosis (Araoz, 1981a) becomes effective, as mentioned in Chapter Four.

INADEQUATE PLEASURE

Because of the greater openness about sexual activities in our society, people, and especially women as a group, expect more of sex than they did in previous generations. Therefore, a careful evaluation is in order to be sure that the expectations are not mythical. Inadequate pleasure covers a continuum, including: mild forms of dissatisfaction with one's sexual response ("I know it could be better"); actual anesthesia of the sexual area; and absence of erotic feelings to all or some sorts of sexual stimulation, at times even when all the physiological responses, including orgasmic contractions, are present. The common characteristic is subjective dissatisfaction because the pleasure is absent or inadequate, as in women who climax after brief stimulation and experience their orgasm as weak and with minimal or no erotic pleasure.

F-5 Symptom Manipulation

Never forgetting the need for combining hypnosis with behavioral maneuvers, Kroger's (Kroger and Fezler, 1976) symptom manipulation methods are useful in some of these cases. For instance, a woman without erotic sensations may be encouraged to keep the symptom in the whole area "except for a small portion of it, where you will feel new, pleasant sensations." This is best accomplished after she has been taught to alter perceived sensations such as temperature, size of limbs, arm levitation, etc., by means of mental activities. If she can alter other sensations hypnotically, she realizes that control of her symptom is possible. However, because there may be psychodynamic reasons for the inadequate pleasure, a progressive approach is always advisable.

F-6 Time Distortion

For those women who climax too soon and with too little pleasure (as well as for premature ejaculators), different forms of time distortions are useful so that, after being experienced, they can be transferred to the sexual situation. Thus, a client who complained about this condition ("I've never had a full orgasm and it always comes too soon") was helped to experience time distortions by "dreaming" an elaborate dream for just one minute and then by reviewing all the pleasant events of her life in just 60 seconds. She was told in hypnosis: "Now for the next 60 seconds, you'll be able to enjoy the most fantastic story in a dream-like fashion. The story will be complicated, involved, but clear to you because you will be part of it." Similar words were used for her life review. When dehypnotized, emphasis was made on the fact that the exercise was so long. Then she was rehypnotized and suggestions to prolong the sexual experience were given. I prefer to suggest a progressive lengthening of the sexual experience, allowing the client's subconscious motivation to choose how much longer the experience should be.

In many cases of inadequate sexual pleasure, mental rehearsal techniques, as described in the previous chapter, are effective; frequently, however, the advisability of employing exploratory techniques becomes self-evident.

FINAL COMMENTS

Respectable research has proven that women spontaneously enjoy different types of erotic imagery during sexual behavior. Hariton (1973; Hariton and Singer, 1974) found that normal, well-adjusted, mentally healthy women, having good relationships with their husbands or lovers, frequently produce "thoughts of an imaginary lover" (the most common) to "being made love to by more than one man at a time" (the least common of ten categories). Long gone is Freud's (1908/1962) dictum: "A happy person never phantasizes, only an unsatisfied one" (p. 146), and the early psychoanalytical position which considered fantasy and imagination in sex escapist maneuvers indicative of neurosis (See Hollender, 1963).

What the findings of this research mean is that hypnotic techniques are a way of channeling therapeutically a natural type of mental activity. To integrate hypnosis in a regimen of sex therapy is to make good use of the naturally healing mechanisms of the mind. The techniques presented in this chapter will, it is hoped, open the door for the experienced therapist to new, creative, and exciting techniques which avoid intellectualization, arguments, and "reasons," and go directly to the source of the sexual difficulty, namely, the inner or subconscious mind.

To integrate sexual imagination with suggestions of enjoyment gives dysfunctional women the needed "permission" to activate a mental activity which up until very recently was not socially acceptable for women, as Hariton (1973) points out. Because of cultural bias about woman's inferiority to man regarding sexual stimulation, particularly visual (an idea reinforced in part by research such as that of Kinsey et al., 1953), the sex therapist must be careful about his/her own possible prejudice in this area. Another pseudo-cultural myth perpetuated by the Freudian penis envy concept, but overwhelmingly contradicted by scientific research (Fisher, 1973) is that of feminine inferiority. The male sex therapist, particularly, has to be vigilantly on guard against it. Finally, as mentioned when dealing with systems theory, because of cultural attitudes it seems to be easier to blame the woman for sexual difficulties in a couple; consequently, the therapist is advised to pay close attention to the systemic interplay between the two partners before isolating the woman as the "identified patient."

8

Hypnotic techniques for male sexual dysfunctions

The outline for this chapter is similar to that of the previous one. Many of the sexual dysfunctions of men come from what Masters and Johnson (1970) described as the almost unbelievable susceptibility of the male to the power of suggestion with regard to his sexual prowess. Because our culture perpetuates the myth of male sexuality (the more the better; never say "No"; always be ready, and so on), men need to become aware of the negative self-hypnosis and cultural expectations that have influenced them from birth. It is interesting to uncover the sexual meaning of so many male attitudes we all take for granted: A man is supposed *to be hard*, never a *softy*, the *bigger* the better; a man should *hold on* to his job and a lot of other things; he is to be energetic, decisive, aggressive. No wonder so many men have sexual problems and feel so despondent when they do!

As in the chapter on women, only the most common dysfunctions will be covered, i.e., vasocongestive dysfunction (erectile problems), dysorgasmia (premature ejaculation, retarded or absent ejaculation), dyspareunia, and inadequate pleasure.

135

VASOCONGESTIVE DYSFUNCTION (VCD)

To stress the parallel between male and female sexual dysfunctions and to move away from the cultural obsession with erection, I prefer to describe erectile problems in physiological terms. Remembering that erectile problems may be the early symptoms of endocrinological malfunctions (as Goldman, 1981, warns) or of diabetes (according to Deutsch and Sherman, 1981), it is essential to be especially careful in the diagnosis. Assuming, therefore, that there is medical clearance and that the VCD is psychogenic, the following hypnotic techniques have been used effectively (Crasilneck and Hall, 1975; Kroger, 1977).

The first method is similar to F-1 (dynamic sexual imagery). After obtaining information about what specific sexual stimuli excite him, the client is helped to relax (see technique T-2 in Chapter Six). Once he is relaxed, a positive imagogic revivification of a happy, peaceful, *nonsexual* scene is introduced, according to information obtained before hypnosis. Let's assume that the client has chosen a beach as his tranquil preference. The therapist will help him to experience himself in a beautiful and safe secluded beach, enjoying every detail: a warm and mild sun, a caressing breeze, the rhythmic movement of the waves, a fantastically blue sky, immaculately white sand, the distant cry of a seagull in the sky, and so on. The man really experiences all these sensations in his mind while enjoying the relaxation.

Once this scene is fully built up, a very attractive but non-threatening woman (his wife or lover or someone else, according to the information obtained pre-hypnotically) is introduced as coming towards him from the distance. If any tension builds up, the woman may turn around and walk away or she may just stand looking at the water. If there is no tension produced by the presence of the woman, she is depicted as friendly, interested in the client, relaxed and relaxing, exciting, etc. (according to his needs). While she is with him in fantasy, he becomes very aroused sexually and experiences an enjoyable, strong erection (all in his imagination) while in trance.

This imagogic scene is made as vivid and realistic as possible and is progressively carried (in two or three sessions, usually) to satisfactory sexual completion, with emphasis on the enjoyment of the erotic experience. The post-hypnotic suggestions are to recreate this fantasy at a given signal, for instance when he touches his wife or lover while naked. Emphasis is placed on the positive sensations of the erection —strong, lasting and pleasurable—which he just enjoys without having to think about it. The wife or sexual partner should share in this hypnotic experience as much as possible.

M-1 Finger Catalepsy

This technique consists in associating a rather common hypnotic behavior, namely that of induced limb catalepsy, with penile erection. First, the client is asked to choose one finger to represent his penis. Then, by vividly imagining that finger becoming like steel, hypnotic catalepsy is achieved. Once this is the case, the comments to the client in trance run along these or similar lines: "As your finger has become now rigid, stiff and hard . . . so your penis will feel more and more rigid and stiff and hard when it's erect. Erect and hard, like your finger, like steel, but alive and feeling and enjoying . . . the pulse . . . making it harder and stiffer and livelier. It'll be such a pleasant surprise . . .you'll be aghast to feel your penis like a mast . . . you'll have a blast . . . your finger, your penis, your mast. Pleasure, joy, peace" (Tilton, 1981).

The post-hypnotic suggestions should establish the connection between the presence of the wife or lover in a sexual situation and the enjoyment of the erection.

Many other techniques can be applied to erectile problems; ego-enhancing methods are especially helpful because of the psychological damage which erectile problems usually produce.

M-2 Arm Levitation

Because of the double symbolism of the arm "going up" in the air and this being produced by a mental activity, this time-honored hypnotic phenomenon may be adapted to VCD in men. Arm levitation may be combined with ego state concepts, by stating, for instance, that "your inner mind, a real part of you, is making your right arm so light and buoyant that you don't have to worry about keeping it so light and buoyant, as if it had a life of its own. It's so nice to feel it going up, getting up. What your inner mind can do when you let it! . . . And you can let your inner mind do this again and again, not just with your arm . . . getting up, staying up . . . it's fun, it feels good . . . right is up . . . and up is right. . . . It'll be right to be up and stay up, without thinking about it with your conscious mind . . . because your inner mind can do it . . . right . . . now."

NLP
can
red

DYSORGASMIA

I prefer the term "dysorgasmia," not too frequently used, to comprise all the ejaculatory dysfunctions: premature, retarded, absent and retrograde. However, we must keep in mind that retrograde or absence of ejaculation has been considered for centuries a feat enhancing sexual pleasure *(coitus reservatus)* or improving the man's intellectual capacity, as some yogis and Chinese teachers believed (Tannahill, 1980), while simultaneously avoiding impregnation.

Regarding prematurity, since self-taught cognitive tricks (non-erotic thoughts) are common among these clients, creating a new type of stress reaction, hypno-relaxation procedures with ego-enhancing techniques are useful. Because many premature ejaculators complain of the absence of erotic sensations as they approach climax, according to Kaplan (1974), they need to regain control of bodily sensations. Paradoxically, then, the following technique (M-3) makes them aware of differences in sensations which they can experience at will.

The medical complications of some male dysorgasmic symptoms are real, especially in retarded or absent ejaculation. These medical complications range from renal failure through abuse of drugs such as narcotics, through gonorrhea or neurological disorders, to post-surgical sequelae. Because of this, all sex therapists must be extremely cautious when the only symptom is retarded or absent ejaculation. This is not to state that psychological factors may not be involved in many cases of retarded or absent ejaculation. It is meant only to emphasize the need for careful differential diagnosis and medical consultation.

M-3 Finger Numbness

For premature ejaculation, by far the most frequent dysorgasmic complaint in men, a helpful technique, besides the positive imagogic experience and the hypnorelaxation described above, is finger numbness. In the category of the transfer techniques (see Chapter Six), it consists in helping the client experience numbness and insensitivity in one finger through hypnotic suggestion and imagery. As in technique M-1, the finger representing his penis is focused on and, through suggestion and imagery, numbness is accomplished and tested. Then, a signal is arranged to recover the ordinary sensations. This signal can be to blink twice in succession or to press the left index finger and thumb together.

Then, the transfer to the penis is effected with the post-hypnotic suggestion that next time he copulates, his penis will feel like his finger feels now: numb and anesthesized. But, still, he will hold a strong erection (feeling happy and enjoying himself), which will last during intercourse as long as he wants. Only when he uses the previous signal, all the normal erotic sensations will return to his penis and he will be able to ejaculate with great pleasure. He has the key to pleasure at his fingertip.

It should be remembered, once more, that sex hypnotherapy also employs the more traditional therapeutic techniques, so that the above procedure is not used as a substitute for such interventions as the squeeze technique, the stop and go technique and others, but in conjunction or sequentially with them.

M-4 Finger Hypersensitivity

For retarded or absent ejaculation, the opposite transfer technique (in conjunction with other behavioral interventions) is to be used. Once the client has entered into hypnosis, hypersensitivity is produced in one finger, choosing the one selected by the client to represent his penis, as before. A signal is also devised, as explained above, to restore the ordinary sensations to the finger. Finally, the transfer of hypersensitivity to the penis, especially to the glans, is effected, with post-hypnotic suggestions similar to the ones for technique M-3.

CASE STUDY

Excerpts from actual therapy sessions may illustrate the clinical use of
the above mentioned techniques. The client, Glenn, a 36-year-old la-
borer, complained about VCD *and* prematurity; however, he claimed
that at some other times he was unable to ejaculate, even after prolonged intercourse. This condition had started after his divorce, five
years previously; he did not experience it during the eight years of his
marriage or before. Glenn had been in a sex group therapy program
for seven months. Though there had been remarkable improvement
during the first month, the problem returned thereafter and "seems to
be even worse than before," as he stated.

After finding out which elements in the first therapy experience had
helped him in any way, these were kept as part of the hypnotherapy.
These were mostly cognitive elements, namely, to realize that many
other men had sexual problems, to know that this can be cured, etc.
Also, it helped him to use relaxation skills when he was becoming
anxious.

At the time he started sex hypnotherapy, he had recently broken
off a relationship which had started very well but had become over-
bearing to him. Consequently, he felt a new sense of relief and freedom. He had just started to date and had engaged in casual sex three
times (each time with a different woman), experiencing VCD in two
cases, and lack of ejaculation in the third. In the first two cases, after
much stimulation, there had been an erection followed by premature
ejaculation. When Glenn started therapy he felt so despondent that
he was talking about suicide.

After the depression was dealt with, his sexual functioning became
the focus of attention. Hypnotic relaxation (namely, relaxation accompanied by non-threatening imagery) was practiced and prescribed
for home use. Also, in the first session, anxiety-free sexual functioning was connected with the relaxation. Glenn was instructed to see
himself in a sexual situation with a very non-threatening woman and
enjoying being flaccid. He was told to allow himself to think of his new
sexual scene (since for Glenn sex without intercourse did not count)
as a make-believe story. Interspersed in the guided sexual imagery
were comments about feeling alive when relaxed, life stirring in his
body, sexual excitement as life, and so on.

Techniques M-1, M-2, M-3 and M-4 were applied in rapid succession and post-hypnotic suggestions regarding his feeling better were given. The whole session lasted almost two full hours.

A week later Glenn arrived on time feeling much better. He had had no dates: The woman he had planned on seeing had gotten sick at the last minute. He had faithfully practiced relaxation every day. Mental rehearsal was used again, together with the previous four "M" techniques. Also, cartoon-like visualization of the control centers in his brain was introduced, so he could "set the dials" that control erections and ejaculations (see Chapter Nine, A-1 technique). Finally, he was invited to remember vividly the pleasant sexual scene of the first session, "as if you had really experienced it, knowing now that sex without intercourse is also okay." It was made clear that he would continue to practice the relaxation exercises alone.

The third session occurred a week later. He had gone out three times with the new woman who had been sick the week before. Twice they ended up in bed together: Glenn had felt much more relaxed, had paid little attention to his performance, and had been much more aware of his feeling of general well-being and pleasure, of his sensations throughout his body. He had experienced satisfying erections. Once they had sexual intercourse. But the second time, Glenn decided to bring her to climax orally and manually and, then, for him to reach orgasm through fellatio. He was feeling great and "cured" and wanted to quit, since he had passed his own test.

He was told to continue practicing self-hypnosis in the form of relaxation exercises, and the techniques of the second session were repeated with more emphasis on his ability to control the functioning of his body. An appointment was made for two weeks later.

Fourth session (two weeks later): He had dated two new women and gone out once more with the woman of two weeks before. Coitus had taken place twice, both times to his satisfaction ("though I know I can be better"). One of the two times had been especially successful: He had reached orgasm once by choice through fellatio, but then he felt aroused once more and—still relaxed and at ease—had intercourse to his satisfaction.

He had continued to practice self-hypnosis every day. The session was used to reinforce the gains made. Before leaving, he was asked whether it was important for him to know and understand what the reasons for his five-year symptom and for his recent cure were. His response was typical of sex hypnotherapy clients: "I thought this is what I've been doing. What do you mean, understand? I know what happened. I saw my divorce as a failure and I was paying for it. I paid enough already . . . although now, I don't see the divorce as a failure."

At the fifth session (two weeks later) Glenn reported continued gains, especially in his relaxed, pleasure-oriented, attitude. He had experienced once what previously he would have considered a failure, "But now, it doesn't bother me. I think of the dials (A-1 technique), of my finger getting stiff, numb or funny, and that ends the crap." More reinforcement through directed self-hypnosis filled the therapy hour. No further appointments were made but a month later Glenn called on the phone to say that everything was going all right and that he was delighted with the progress made. He was told to buy Zilbergeld's (1978) book on male sexuality (which was just out), but not to read anything in it until a month later. Then he was told to read only Chapter Four, which deals with the ten male sexual myths, and to take as long as he needed in reading it. It was emphatically stated that this was part of the sex therapy program and that not to follow these directions carefully could undo all the good done so far. Only after reading Chapter Four was he allowed to read any other part of the book. The rationale for this injunction was to provide some source of anxiety related with sex, in case there was some psychological need to have it. Also, it gave Glenn a chance to continue to improve his sexual attitude and to have a source book for further questions or doubts.

In the next year, Glenn referred two other men for treatment. Since I was interested in the final outcome of this client in order to report it in this book, I called him two years after termination. This follow up was also positive and confirmed the gains made.

DYSPAREUNIA

The etiology of male dyspareunia is mostly organic (Wear, 1976), though psychological factors, such as the anticipation of pain, are present in some cases (Sharpe and Meyer, 1973). This means that the sex therapist must obtain all relevant information for an accurate diagnosis, such as degree of lubrication of the woman, use of contraceptive devices or artificial lubricants, previous genital surgery of the woman or, obviously, congenital anomalies in her. On the part of the man, abnormal anatomical conditions of the penis, as well as infections and irritations, may cause pain in intercourse.

If the man experiences pain in ejaculation, rather than in copulation, it may be an indication of prostate or other internal inflammatory conditions which require medical attention. Once there is medical attendance, hypnosis can be used for dyspareunia as it is used in any other form of pain control (Hilgard and Hilgard, 1975). A transfer approach, from an anesthetized hand to the area of pain, is effective and simple, as is a modification of the A-1 technique. In the latter case, imaginary dials controlling sensitivity are set carefully, so that the person experiences sensations but no pain.

INADEQUATE PLEASURE

As in the case of women (see Chapter Seven) this is usually a rather generalized and vague presenting problem: "I feel nothing during sex." "My mind wanders and I end up exhausted from the sheer mental effort of concentrating." "It's okay, but I know it's not half as good as it used to be", etc. It should be remembered that the man experiences no difficulty with his body: Arousal, erection, ejaculation—all are normal. His subjective feelings of pleasure and satisfaction, however, are lacking.

In men, too, one may visualize a continuum or a scale to help clients report on their inadequate pleasure. The therapist must examine closely how satisfying *the relationship* is, if there is one, and realize that, though the presenting complaint may be sexual, the real problem may be relational.

Assuming that the difficulty is, indeed, inadequate sexual pleasure, those techniques listed for female dyspareunia (F-5, F-6) are effective. Two other techniques are discussed below.

M-5 Becoming Alive

Similar to P-3 (wellness), this technique centers on the forces of life in the individual. The client is guided through a detailed awareness of sensations (his breathing, heart beat, weight of hands on lap or arm rests, pressure of buttocks and back on chair, etc.). He is asked to let each physical part become fully alive, to increase the sensations as one does with the volume of a radio. Then, after he has accomplished this successfully, he may focus on his testicles and penis, also feeling them very alive. Some clients become very good at this and soon are aware of their pulse in different parts of their bodies. The therapist may use the pulse (or breathing itself) to bring to the client the awareness of life and living: "Your body is alive, but life is not always loud and noisy. You are listening now to the hush of life in you. Get more in touch with your life; experience it more in your legs (or other area). Rejoice in the life that flows through you, in you; enjoy the life that is you. Now let it gush into your testicles and penis, filling them — you — fully alive." The post-hypnotic suggestions are directed to the next sexual situation: "Life making itself felt in me, with pleasure. Life and pleasure, one, together, when I am with my wife (or lover)," etc.

As has been stated before, there is no reason to limit oneself to only one hypnotic technique in the same session. After the sex therapist has mastered these techniques, combining two or more techniques becomes the natural thing to do in clinical practice.

M-6 Mental Exaggeration

The man in hypnosis is encouraged to mentally represent, in a cartoon-like fashion, the most pleasurable and fun-filled sexual experience he could possibly have. Once he starts getting into it, all inner senses that apply should be involved, so that the mental representation becomes a real "experience." The pleasure in his internal representation becomes then so exaggerated that he wants to tone it down.

This process of increasing pleasure to the point that it is too much, in order to weaken it to a comfortable level, is then repeated several times with suggestions that too much pleasure can become uncomfortable and he may have to tone it down in sex eventually.

FINAL COMMENTS

Pietropinto and Simenauer (1977), among others, have shown that many men feel basically insecure sexually. That is one reason for the frequent use of reaction formation as a defensive technique to hide that insecurity. This has to be kept in mind when doing sex therapy for male dysfunctions. Here hypnosis becomes useful for ego enhancement and strengthening in general, before it focuses specifically on the particular sexual dysfunction (Araoz, 1972).

I believe that men feel basically insecure because of three existential realities: the long dependency on the mother, copulation itself, and the reproduction of life. Regarding the first factor, not until the 1940s was there a reliable formula to substitute for the mother's milk. Without a woman, man could not be. And until puberty, women keep influencing his development. The woman has a lot to do regarding the male's sense of self. Man senses that "Woman" has too much control over his life.

The second source of man's sense of insecurity is copulation. By the time of puberty, the boy has centered much of his identity on his penis. But this organ, giving him pride and self-respect, is also man's great vulnerability. The unspeakable fear of "impotence" starts with sexual maturity. In the sexual encounter, the man must "show" his potency. And by the very nature of the act, the woman "takes away" man's power, his erection, and thus it seems as if she can destroy his self.

Finally, the reproduction of life is the third source of man's sense of insecurity. The feverish energy with which man has traditionally tried to change nature and the high technology by which what is can be altered are indications of man's frustration at not being able to produce life himself. On the other hand, the playful joy with which man has engaged in war and destruction since the beginning of history makes us wonder about the psychological motivation underlying such behavior. If he cannot produce life, his way of being on top of it is by destroying it.

Because of these three sources of insecurity, sex hypnotherapy for men should not focus too narrowly on the sexual symptom, but consider the need to reinforce and strengthen the whole personality. The lack of sexual desire in men (see Chapter Nine) often stems from that existential sense of inferiority which, once addressed, improves the whole self-esteem and restores adequate sexual interest and desire.

9

Hypnotic techniques for dysfunctions of sexual desire and processing

The techniques for these two types of sexual problems are grouped together because both of these aspects of human sexuality are intimately connected with "thinking," and because there is no evidence on sex differences in these conditions. Much more needs to be learned about the chemical and physiological processes which might be involved in diminished or absent sexual desire and in negative processing after sexual activity. We are at a point in time when little is definitely known about the somatic components of these sexual dysfunctions and, therefore, I am limiting my discussion to the psychological or mental components of sexual abulia and negativism.

The clinician must be sure that the clients are properly diagnosed and that relational dissatisfaction and other problems are not the real cause of these symptoms.

In disorders of both desire and processing, the presence of negative self-hypnosis must be considered and the procedure suggested in Chapter Four followed. To review briefly, the procedure consists of first uncovering the negative statements and mental imagery about sex that the person is in the habit of accepting or even fostering. The second step is to "positivize" those negative mental activities with ele-

146

ments which are idiosyncratic and ego-syntonic. The third step is to apply hypnotically these positive self-statements and mental images and to keep practicing until the latter become so familiar that the former (negative elements) are extinguished.

Within the framework of counteracting negative self-hypnosis, some of the general techniques listed in Chapter Six are especially useful for these disorders. Among them, ego-states (P-1) and the affect bridge (T-1), the body speaks (E-3) and the message symptom (P-2), as well as ideomotor questioning (D-3) are convenient techniques to keep in mind. An adaptation of F-1 (dynamic sexual imagery) may also be used.

The two main sections of this chapter focus more specifically on particular techniques for desire and for processing disorders.

SEXUAL DESIRE DYSFUNCTION

We simply have no absolute, objective, or prescriptive norm for sexual desire. It is "inadequate" in a purely subjective way, considering the sexual dyad as a system. One member of the dyad may be perfectly pleased with the frequency and quality of sex, while the other is definitely not. This may be enough to diagnose sexual abulia (Araoz, 1980a), inadequate sexual interest (Jehu, 1979), inhibited sexual desire (Lief, 1977), or hypoactive sexual desire (Kaplan, 1979). On the other hand, there are reports of "happy sexless marriages" (Martin, 1977), where the absence of sex is not a matter of distress for those involved in an otherwise satisfying and intimate relationship. However, from all the evidence available, this situation is the exception.

Before proceeding any further, it should be noted that most people experience periods of diminished interest in sex—the cultural myth of perpetual readiness for sex, especially in the male, notwithstanding. Others very rarely, if ever, think of sex themselves, but enjoy it and function without difficulty when a sexual opportunity presents itself or when the partner initiates the encounter. Finally, and still along this varied continuum, one finds those whose sexual abulia is associated with more objectively definable sexual dysfunctions, either of arousal or climax.

Because sexual interest and desire are as subjective as the amount of food intake, or the number of hours used for sleep, the clinician's perception has to be free from personal contaminations. There is nothing "wrong" with many variations of sexual interest and desire. Nevertheless, when a person reports a recent change in the pattern without significant change in the relationship or in the general circumstances of life, it is wise to consider the possibility of organic factors needing medical attention. There is not necessarily a direct relationship between, for instance, a general systemic illness or an endocrine disorder and diminished or absent sexual desire, but the possibility is there. In some cases, the disorder of sexual desire may be one of the first indications of physical illness.

The hypnotic techniques to be described assume that the sexually abulic person is *not* having other problems, either relational, occupational, or medical.

A-1 The Inner Dials

In a cartoon-like or animated fashion, the person who is in hypnosis is invited to visualize the interior of his/her mind as the central control room of a highly sophisticated computer. There the client is to hear the buzzing of the machinery, recognize the typical smell of a computer room, watch the flashing lights on the switches and panels, feel the temperature in the room, and perceive any other sensations. Once the client is really getting into this inner daydream-like reality, the clinician suggests that one of the dials controls sexual desire. The dial is "seen" clearly: It has numbers from 0 to 10; there is a soft blue color in the area of the lower numbers which gradually becomes an intense red in the number 10 zone. The person is to examine this dial carefully and note a knob to control its needle directly below the dial. The client is encouraged to set the dial for the right number and to be sure that the needle stays there, with only half a point of play on either side of the number chosen.

The post-hypnotic suggestions refer to this inner reality so that the person has all the good feelings belonging to this level of sexual desire whenever the situation requires it. The client is also encouraged to practice this many times on his/her own.

A-2 Revivification

The goal of this technique is to relive a period in the person's life when sexual functioning was exciting and desired. For this, a very good sexual experience of one's past is chosen and built in detail, helping the client become keenly aware of all positive and pleasurable sensations, as has been done in other techniques, such as (F-1) dynamic sexual imagery. The post-hypnotic suggestions emphasize the good feelings, sense of enjoyment, and happiness which will be present when a sexual opportunity presents itself.

However, when the individual has no memory of a satisfying sexual experience (as in the clinical vignette which follows), the client will be encouraged to "make up" a sexual fantasy that becomes desirable. As explained in Chapter Four, in the section on Therapeutic Hypnosis, s/he may also be asked to imagine his/her favorite "sex symbol" in an exciting sexual scene. After several mental exercises with that sex symbol in focus, the client may slowly substitute him/herself in the mental picture. Depending on the level of anxiety, it might be necessary to have the client imagine (after working with the favorite sex symbol) first *a movie* of him/herself, before "stepping into the movie," as it were, and allowing full enjoyment of the sexual fantasy.

A CLINICAL VIGNETTE

This case of lack of sexual desire was quite different from the case of Jim, reported elsewhere (Araoz, 1980a). Marilu was 36, had been married ten years and had three children, ages 9, 7, and 5½. She had been the oldest and brightest child in a family of seven siblings and at the age of 15 had entered a convent to become a Roman Catholic nun, resigning eight years later. She went into nursing school and had no dates or hetero- or homosexual behavior until she became a nurse. Then, she started to go out with a friend of her father, a wealthy businessman, 17 years her senior, who "wanted to have a family." She married him when she was 26. Until her marriage, Marilu had been a virgin, non-passionate kissing being all the affectionate behavior she and her future husband had engaged in during the six months of courtship. Her husband, "understanding and loving," had treated her like a child initially and had considered sex only for reproduction. He had shown no interest in sex whatsoever, which fitted well with Marilu, who had agreed with the reproductive view of sex as its only purpose.

However, in the last year things had changed. Marilu's husband had rearranged his business so that he could retire at the age of 52 and, since his retirement, had become interested in sex. According to Marilu, this had been a sudden and radical change—practically no sex in nine years of marriage, and now during the last 12 months, "all he wants is to make love, to read and watch erotic stuff, as if he were just obsessed with it."

He explained this change in terms of his new outlook on life since his retirement. He had worked hard all his life, he had attained all his goals, and more. Now he wanted to enjoy and pay attention to the areas he had previously neglected, especially sex. He had come to the realization that his former view of sex had been too narrow and was determined to have a good time. He loved his wife and did not believe in extramarital relations.

Marilu had tried to accommodate him, but was just not interested. Sex, for her, was still a duty and, much as she tried, she was unable to look forward to it. However, she admitted that "once I'm into it, I don't mind it." But arguments and fights developed inevitably, especially at the planning stage of any special trip. The husband wanted them to go away by themselves in their yacht without the children. She didn't mind leaving the children because they had trustworthy housekeepers and maids. But she knew that going away alone meant many opportunities for sex and so the children had become the excuse for not going and the bone of contention.

In the first visit to me, Marilu kept talking about "doing what is right" and pleasing her husband. I talked about learning new means of enjoying sex for herself, not just out of duty or love for her husband. With the husband's enthusiastic approval, it was agreed that Marilu could initiate sex and express her desire for sex, and that this behavior did not mean that she was not feminine. She admitted that she had never had desire for sex and had never initiated it. No further discussion was encouraged, but the possibility of learning more about sex was proposed. Once she had agreed "to learn" new aspects of sex, we started by studying her negative self-hypnosis. In her case, negativism was not directed principally at sex but at her husband's behavior. In spite of her sexual abulia, Marilu was not sexophobic. She was quick to identify negative affirmations ("There must be something wrong with him") and imagery (visualizing his face while in erotic passion as some kind of psychotic facial distortion).

The next step was to "positivize" the previous mental activity and then use it hypnotically. Again, it was not difficult for Marilu, based on her previous statement regarding her good feelings once she got into sex, to construct a pleasure hierarchy. This consisted of a list of items in her sexual experience with her husband which she found even slightly more pleasurable than others. Marilu reported this sequence:

(1) To be held in an embrace and to feel his skin against hers.

(2) To feel the pressure of his chest against her breasts.

(3) To feel his erect penis pressing on her thighs.

(4) To feel his penis inside her vagina.

This hierarchy served for the progressive method of self-hypnosis, with Marilu using these items and repeating to herself how good, beautiful, peaceful, and fulfilling each one of these sensations was.

From this the sexual mental scene was enriched further until she found his passion beautiful and exciting (not fearful, as before) and their mutual sexual experience 100 percent positive.

Two post-hypnotic suggestions were given: First, that the good feelings experienced in hypnosis would return when she and her husband were in the bedroom, ready to retire. Marilu needed a sense of control of the new desire for sex, so that to experience those feelings *before* being in bed gave her time to decide whether to act on them or not. The second post-hypnotic suggestion was that the whole chain of reactions culminating in a clear, enjoyable desire for sex would be elicited by her husband's naked embrace. Consequently, she could refuse his embrace when she did not want to act on her sexual desire, or, on the other hand, she could initiate the embrace when she wanted to act on those new feelings. In other words, the new sexual desire would not control her unless she wanted it.

After four weeks of practicing this type of mental exercise, the couple reported great improvement, and Marilu herself admitted joyfully that now she had found herself spontaneously thinking of sex as fun together, and wanting it. The couple was seen every other week for two more months, during which period the gains made became solidified.

SEXUAL PROCESSING DYSFUNCTIONS

Negative processing (see Chapter Four) is the mental activity, mostly subconscious, connected with any aspect of sex leading to guilt, anxiety, or anger. Similar to certain forms of tension, detected by biofeedback equipment but not on the awareness range of the individual, negative processing is recognized most often by its effects. The origin of negative processing is varied, namely, cultural myths, religious injunctions (what Kroger, 1977, has called "ecclesiological neurosis"), personal history, and experience.

The problem with sexual cultural myths was discussed in Chapter Five. The second category may require the collaboration of a religious leader who, in cooperation with the sex therapist, "gives permission" to the client to feel or act in a sexual manner. The individual's personal history and experience, covering unhappy previous dating to victimization in cases of rape or incest, may require more traditional psychotherapy before sex therapy, as such, is employed. However, even in the last category, and while the person is receiving psychotherapy, I have found that simultaneous sex hypnotherapy is beneficial. In some cases, the latter accelerates and shortens the psychotherapy.

Although the consequences of negative sexual processing are many, I am limiting my discussion to *guilt, anger,* and *anxiety* because these are the most common and pervasive, leading the person to lack of sexual desire and to sexual avoidance. These three feelings are seldom distinctly isolated; in each case, however, it is easy to find the prevalence of either guilt, anger, or anxiety. The hypnotic techniques that follow address themselves to this prevalence. As I mentioned before, negative processing is negative self-hypnosis applied specifically to sexual behavior and it may take place prior to, during, and/or after the sexual engagement.

Before presenting specific techniques for cases where guilt, anger, or anxiety is prevalent, the following general hypnotic techniques are offered for all cases of negative processing.

H-1 True Statements

Many people who engage in negative processing know intellectually what is right about sex. After listing as a couple the "true statements", one or more important authority figures are identified, that is, historical or living people considered authorities by the client. The client is asked whether they would agree with those "true" statements about sex. Then, the client enters hypnosis. When the alternate state of awareness has been reached, one of these authority figures (or all of them in unison) is pictured lecturing or preaching along the ideas of the true statements about sex. The mental picture is made very vivid. The "authority" is teaching the client, not anybody. However, others, such as parents and early teachers who might have conveyed wrong or negative sexual concepts, may also be in "the audience," listening to the lecture. This should end with a powerful exhortation to act accordingly and to do what is right sexually. The "authority" must be seen as telling the client what it means to let negative feelings ruin a healthy, natural, and enjoyable experience.

It should be noted that some people actually believe that everything about sex is sinful, wrong, and to be avoided. In this case, direct sex education is needed, with the cooperation of any respected religious or moral authority. However, in these exceptional cases who request therapy, the relationship is often the issue (what is the meaning of this deep antagonism in a relationship?) to be resolved before the sexual interaction is examined.

In other cases, the negative processing is limited to something "wrong" in an otherwise accepted sexual interaction. Thus, one finds, for instance, men, repulsed by the labia or by cunnilingus, or women negative about the penis or fellatio—in general, any sexual fears, at times reaching the severity of a phobia. If the clients want to overcome this negative reaction (in other words, if they don't intellectually believe these to be truly wrong), the following technique may be employed.

H-2 The Artist Within

Once in hypnosis, the client is encouraged to change the previous negative image to a poetic one. Thus, for instance, the labia may appear as a beautiful flower or a precious sea shell; the vagina as an exciting and safe underground cave; the penis as a magnificent ivory ornament. Oral contact may be seen as a unique form of communion, similar to kissing a religious symbol or image.

In this technique, as has been mentioned repeatedly before, all inner senses must be engaged, building up the positive mental representation as richly as possible.

The clinical rationale for this mental exercise (even when another form of therapy is simultaneously administered) is the need to have a new skill to stop the negative imagery associated with specific sexual areas or activities.

It goes without saying that in this case, the previous technique of appealing to authority (H-1) may also be helpful.

H-3 Reeducating the Inner Child

When the negative mental processing produces mostly feelings of *guilt*, it may be helpful to trace its origins and to remember the early scenes where guilt was associated with sex. Then, in hypnosis, the client sees him/herself as a child in those scenes, experiencing the many sensations and feelings related to them. When this is accomplished, the adult self, as it looks in the present, is introduced into the mental picture and is encouraged to use all his/her current resources, wisdom, and understanding to "bring up the inner child" without neurotic guilt, to encourage the inner child to recognize the real distinction between right and wrong and to have clear ideas about the body, its functions, and pleasure.

The same type of exercise may have to be repeated at different ages in the client's development, when guilt-ridden messages were received. The adult self may have to help the inner child to forgive those who gave the negative messages or to excuse their motivation.

This technique has helped many guilt-ridden clients to change negative into positive processing.

H-4 Wear Out the Anger

Using one of the uncovering techniques (see Chapter Six), the origin of the connection between sex and *anger* is usually quickly discovered. Some clients report that they feel angry when they think of having sex, while they do, or after the sexual encounter. This particular outcome is frequently an indication of unresolved relational problems going back to very early stages of development. Psychotherapy is indicated in most of these cases. In conjunction with it, the therapist may want to keep this hypnotic technique in mind.

When the person is in hypnosis, s/he is asked to experience the anger as something like a volcano, a mighty river, a fire, an earthquake, or the like. Once the idiosyncratic mental image has subconsciously been chosen and experienced with all possible intensity, it is allowed to develop and wear itself out.

Then, a mental picture of sex without anger is encouraged. If this does not happen, this is a good indication of the need for psychotherapy. If it does occur, the contrast is emphasized and statements like these are expressed: "It will be so good to *enjoy* sex. Whatever caused that anger in the past can stay in the past. The anger can consume itself and give way to something new, fresh, strong, and healthy. Without that (volcano, fire, earthquake, or whatever), sex can be enjoyment. Sex and peace; sex and good feelings, while you enjoy the scenery without (the volcano or fire or whatever). Get into those feelings: quiet, peace, harmony, joy," and so on, along these lines.

Finally, in some cases, the habitual outcome of negative processing is *anxiety*. As in the other two instances mentioned previously, exploratory techniques often prove beneficial. Also, relaxation (as in T-2) is extremely helpful because often these people, through years of unconscious practice, have conditioned themselves to associate sex with feelings of anxiety.

Besides the above, a specific hypnotic technique (developed by Bleck, 1981) for this condition is offered to the clinician as a sample, so that s/he may construct new ones with the same goal of dissociating the thought of sex from anxiety.

H-5 The Movie Director

In hypnosis, the client is encouraged "to see" him/herself in the exact same sexual circumstances which elicit all the anxiety. As in previous techniques, the anxious scene is built up with all possible details. Once the client has captured this anxiety-provoking scene, s/he is told to become the movie director for this scene and to change it in any way possible to make it less anxious, or even completely anxiety-free.

This is repeated several times with the suggestions that "You are the director, you control the situation, you are changing it right now." The post-hypnotic suggestions refer to reliving "the good scene" when the opportunity presents itself.

In cases when negative sexual processing produces mostly anxiety (rather than guilt or anger), relaxation and mental rehearsal techniques cannot be ignored.

A CASE OF NEGATIVE SEXUAL PROCESSING

Mick, 27, and Pearl, 29, had been living together for three years. Mick had been married before. During the process of divorce, she had met Pearl and, after several months, recognized that her sexual orientation had always been homosexual. About a year later, they moved in together. Their presenting problem was tension between them, centered on the fact that Mick had not told her family about her relationship with Pearl. This was causing discomfort when Mick visited her family, since she felt they suspected their homosexuality.

Soon it became clear that the real problem was their poor sexual relationship, not the issue with Mick's family—which they could handle by themselves. Both Pearl and Mick had been raised in strict religious families. Homosexuality was condemned as sinful. But Pearl's family had accepted her as gay. However, she still believed there was something wrong with her. Initially, both thought Mick's negative thinking ruined their sexual enjoyment. But after focusing on possible elements of negative processing, feelings of guilt, anxiety, and anger emerged as regular concomitants of their sexual experiences and even of their individual thoughts.

After use of H-1 (true statements), H-3 (reeducating the inner child), and H-5 (the movie director) several times during the first session and suggestions that they practice at home, quick changes started to take place. Both Pearl and Mick reported "more fun and less tension" one week later at the second hypnotherapy session. Mick had been distracted while practicing alone, but had been "really into it" when doing self-hypnosis together with Pearl. The same techniques were practiced repeatedly in the second session and the injunction of practicing at home every day, if possible, was repeated. The next visit had to be scheduled three weeks later.

They had practiced 15 times in 21 days and they were delighted with their progress. Mick said that only once had she felt some "shadow of guilt" during the last three weeks. Their mutual sexual activities had increased, and there was a generally lighter atmosphere, more playfulness between them.

A third session was conducted as a follow-up two weeks later, during which ego-strengthening messages were stronger than before. It was agreed not to schedule another session, but that they would call for an appointment if they needed it. Two months later, Pearl called to say "Hello," reporting that everything was much better and that the relationship was stronger than ever before.

As some sort of a footnote, I'd like to add an interesting anecdote connected with this case. These two women had two friends, a gay couple, who were also having sexual problems. They told me that they were thinking of teaching them how to use hypnosis. I explained why this should not be done, namely, the unexpected material from subconscious levels that can emerge in hypnosis and the need for specialized training to handle these situations.

As professionals, we teach self-hypnosis for an individual person's benefit or (in most cases of sexual dysfunctions) for the individual couple's enrichment. Our message must come through very clearly that we are *not* teaching them a mental skill that may be used indiscriminately. We do not need to request the signing of a legal document in which they promise to use hypnosis only on themselves. But we should not assume that all clients understand how to use this new method unless we take our time to explain our position against people non-trained in psychology, psychotherapy, and psychopathology using hypnosis on others for therapeutic purposes.

FINAL COMMENTS

In Chapters Six through Nine, I have described almost 40 hypnotic techniques for sex therapy. To repeat what was stated before: Though superficially they may look like a list of food recipes, they are intended for the seasoned sex therapist who, after an initial exposure to hypnosis, wants to apply the latter clinically. They are also meant for other mental health workers who may be well versed in hypnosis but want therapeutic approaches for sexual dysfunctions as such.

No therapeutic technique, hypnotic or otherwise, has value in itself. There is no *ex opere operato* or sacramental efficacy in any of these interventions and in no way do I want to convey even the semblance of such "force." Each one of these techniques makes sense only in the context of a therapeutic relationship, fulfilling the conditions of *empathy, warmth* (including acceptance), and *genuineness,* as extensive studies (Mitchell et al., 1977), based on earlier Rogerian research (Truax and Carkhuff, 1967), have shown. Only in a context of "interactive collaboration between patient and hypnotherapist, along with respect for the patient's autonomy," to quote Fromm (1981), can techniques acquire human meaning. The indiscriminate application of techniques is technology, but sex hypnotherapy (like any other form of genuine intervention *to help the client grow and develop one's potential, beyond one's self-imposed limitations*) requires these three qualities of genuineness, warmth, and empathy. These, assuming scientific knowledge of human behavior, move therapy from technology to art.

The two clinical cases presented in this chapter tried to convey flexibility, readiness to change course, and constant respect for the clients, as well as the attitude that the therapist does not necessarily know what is best for the client. Nevertheless, the therapist's duty is to know how to go about finding out what is best for the client and how to help the client attain what is best for him or her.

Conclusions

"It is the task of the therapist to enrich the patient, to help expand the ego span and to give pride in the ability to cope and master" (Fromm, 1981, p. 427).

These words sum up my belief in the goals of psychotherapy. Because they are written specifically in an article on the values of hypnotherapy they are of special interest. In sex hypnotherapy, therefore, one takes a natural, elegant and parsimonious approach. It is natural because people are taught to use their mind in ways neglected by them earlier. It is elelgant because the route to the problem's answer is direct and thus the problem is simplified. Finally, it is a parsimonious and economical approach in that it encourages self-therapy by insisting on the need to practice alone and as a couple what is learned in the consulting room, actively involving the clients in their own move to wellness. Thus, the goals mentioned above are fulfilled.

By teaching clients self-hypnosis, I am encouraging self-help. This is no endorsement whatsoever of clients becoming hypnotherapists for others on the basis of their personal use of hypnosis. But it is an opportunity for most to start viewing themselves differently and in a healthier light. They are no longer prisoners of their own negative self-hypnosis, but they become free through the mastery of mental resources of which they were only vaguely aware before. This inner ability is generally extended quite spontaneously to other areas in their lives, so that starting from their sexual problem they start feeling more "potent" in interpersonal relations, in their work, in their whole *Weltanschauung*.

More and more evidence converges on the fact that self-hypnosis is as natural as reverie (Singer and Pope, 1981). By teaching sex therapy clients the skill to use a natural resource of their own, one gives them also a new sense of mastery over themselves and, consequently, a new inner strength. Clients have to be reminded, however, that this is a personal skill to be used on themselves, not on others.

To come back to the therapists for whom this book was written, I have pointed the way to progress from mere sex therapy to sex hypnotherapy. After reviewing all the advantages of hypnosis, it is up to the sex therapist to decide whether s/he wants to become a sex *hypnotherapist*. As has been implied before, no book is sufficient, under ordinary circumstances, to make one feel at ease with the employment of a new therapeutic tool such as hypnosis. The professional, proud of his/her work, will be glad to obtain additional training by reputable instructors sponsored by reputable organizations.

The therapists who, with an open mind, dare look into unfamiliar though proven methods for helping their clients more effectively will reap many personal satisfactions and will, in truth, benefit their charges. Hypnosis has much to offer in sex therapy. Sex therapy is enriched when it becomes sex hypnotherapy.

References

AHSEN, A. Image for effective psychotherapy: An essay on consciousness, anticipation and imagery. In A. A. Sheikh & J. T. Shaffer (Eds.), *The Potential of Fantasy and Imagination.* New York: Brandon House, 1979.

ARAOZ, D. L. Male inferiority. *Sexual Behavior,* 1972, 2, 7, 34.

ARAOZ, D. L. Review of *The New Sex Therapy,* by H. S. Kaplan. *Journal of Family Counseling,* 1975, 3, 2, 75-77.

ARAOZ, D. L. Clinical hypnosis in couple therapy. *Journal of the American Society of Psychosomatic Dentistry and Medicine,* 1978, 25, 58-67.

ARAOZ, D. L. Hypnocounseling. *Educational Resources Information Center* (ERIC), 1979, ED 182 624.

ARAOZ, D. L. Clinical hypnosis in treating sexual abulia. *American Journal of Family Therapy,* 1980, 8, 1, 48-57 (a).

ARAOZ, D. L. Enriching sex therapy with hypnosis. In H. Wain (Ed.), *Clinical Hypnosis in Medicine.* Chicago: Yearbook Medical Publishers, 1980 (b).

ARAOZ, D. L. Review of *Disorders of Sexual Desire,* by H. S. Kaplan, *American Journal of Family Therapy,* 1980, 8, 3, 83-85 (c).

ARAOZ, D. L. *Role of negative and positive self-hypnosis in sexual functioning.* Paper presented at the 88th Annual Convention of the American Psychological Association, Montreal, September 1980 (d).

ARAOZ, D. L. Negative self-hypnosis. *Journal of Contemporary Psychotherapy,* 1981, 12, 1, 45-51 (a).

ARAOZ, D. L. *Hypnosex: From the job of sex to the joy fo sex.* Paper presented at the annual meeting of the American Society of Clinical Hypnosis, Boston, November 1981 (b).

ARAOZ, D. L. Review of *Sexual Dysfunction: A Behavioral Approach,* by D. Jehu. *American Journal of Family Therapy,* 1981, 9, 2, 98-99 (c).

ARAOZ, D. L. & BLECK, R. T. *Hypnosex.* New York: Arbor House, 1982.

ASCHER, L. M. The role of hypnosis in behavior therapy. *Annals of the N.Y. Academy of Sciences,* 1977, 269, 250-263.

BACH, G. *Illusions.* New York: Dell, 1977.

BANDLER, R. & GRINDER, J. *The Structure of Magic, I.* Palo Alto, CA.: Science & Behavior Book. 1975 (a).

BANDLER, R. & GRINDER, J. *Patterns of the Hypnotic Techniques of M. H. Erickson* (2 vols.). Cupertino, CA.: Meta Publications, 1975 (b).

BANDLER, R. & GRINDER, J. *Frogs into Princes: Neuro-Linguistic Programing.* Moab, Utah: Real People Press, 1979

BANDURA, A. *Principles of Behavior Modification.* New York: Holt, Rinehart & Winston, 1969.
BANDURA, A. Self-efficacy: Towards a unifying theory of behavior change. *Psychological Review,* 1977, 89, 191-215.
BARBACH, L. *Women Discover Orgasm.* New York: Free Press, 1980.
BARBER, T. X. *Hypnosis: A Scientific Approach.* New York: Van Nostrand Reinhold Co., 1969.
BARBER, T. X. *Hypnosis: A Scientific Approach.* New York: Psychological Dimensions, 1976.
BARBER, T. X. *Hypnosis and Psychosomatics.* San Francisco: Proseminar Institute, 1978.
BARBER, T. X. *Self-suggestions for personal growth and the future of hypnosis.* Paper presented at the 88th Annual Convention of the American Psychological Association, Montreal, September 1980.
BARBER, T. X., SPANOS, H. P. & CHAVES, J. F. *Hypnotism: Imagination and Human Potentials.* Elmsford, N.Y.: Pergamon Press, 1974.
BATESON, G. *Steps to an Ecology of Mind.* New York: Ballantine Books, 1972.
BEACH, F. A. (Ed.) *Sex and Behavior.* New York: John Wiley & Sons, 1965.
BEACH, F. A. & FORD, C. S. *Patterns of Sexual Behavior.* New York: Harper Bros., 1951.
BECK, A. T. *Cognitive Therapy and the Emotional Disorders.* New York: International Universities Press, 1976.
BECK, A. T., RUSH, A. J., SHAW, B. F. & EMERY, G. *Cognitive Therapy of Depression: A Treatment Manual.* New York: Guilford, 1979.
BEIGEL, H. G. *Advances in Sex Research,* New York: Harper & Row, 1963.
BEIGEL, H. G. The use of hypnosis in female sexual anesthesia. *Journal of the American Society of Psychosomatic Dentistry and Medicine,* 1972, 19, 4-14.
BERNARD, T. *Hatha Yoga.* London: Rider & Co., 1950.
BERNHEIM, H. M. *Hypnosis and Suggestion in Psychotherapy: A Treatise on the Nature and Uses of Hypnotism* (English translation by C. A. Herter, 1888; reissued by E. R. Hilgard) New Hyde Park, N.Y.: University Books, 1964.
BLECK, R. T. The movie director technique in hypnosis. Personal Communication, September 30, 1981.
BOGEN, I. Sexual myths and politics. *Journal of Sex Education and Therapy,* 1981, 7, 1, 7-15.
BOWEN, M. *Family Therapy in Clinical Practice.* New York: Aronson, 1978.
BOWERS, K. S. *Hypnosis for the Seriously Curious.* Monterey, CA.: Brooks/Cole, 1976.
BOWERS, K. S. Listening with the third ear: On paying inattention effectively. In F. H. Frankel & H. S. Zamansky (Eds.), *Hypnosis at Its Bicentennial.* New York: Plenum, 1978.
BRENMAN, M. & GILL, M. M. *Hypnotherapy.* New York: International Universities Press, 1947.
BROWN, B. B. *Supermind: The Ultimate Energy.* New York: Harper & Row, 1980.
BROWN, J. M. & CHAVES, J. F. Hypnosis in the treatment of Sexual Dysfunction. *Journal of Sex and Marital Therapy,* 1980, 6, 63-74.
BRY, A. *Directing the Movies of Your Mind.* New York: Harper & Row, 1978.
BUTLER, C. A. New data about female sexual response. *Journal of Sex and Marital Therapy,* 1976, 2, 40-46.
CAPRIO, F. S. & BERGER, J. R. *Helping Yourself with Self-Hypnosis.* Englewood Cliffs, N.J.: Prentice-Hall, 1963.
CASTANEDA, C. *Journey to Ixtlan.* New York: Simon & Shuster, 1972.
CASTANEDA, C. *Tales of Power.* New York: Simon & Shuster, 1974.
CAUTELA, J. R. Treatment of compulsive behavior by covert sensitization. *Psychological Record,* 1966, 16, 33-41.
CAUTELA, J. R. Covert sensitization. *Psychological Reports,* 1967, 20, 459-468.
CAUTELA, J. R. Covert reinforcement. *Behavior Therapy,* 1970, 1, 33-50.
CAUTELA, J. R. Covert conditioning. In A. Jacobs and L. B. Sachs (Eds.), *The Psychology of Private Events: Perspectives on Covert Response Systems.* New York: Academic Press, 1971.
CAUTELA, J. R. Covert conditioning in hypnotherapy. *International Journal of Clinical and Ex-*

perimental Hypnosis, 1975, 23, 15-27.

CAUTELA, J. R. Covert conditioning: Assumptions and procedures. *Journal of Mental Imagery,* 1977, 1, 53-64.

CAUTELA, J. R., WALSH, K. & WISH, P. A. The use of covert reinforcement in the modification of attitudes towards the retarded. *Journal of Psychology,* 1971, 77, 257-260.

CHEEK, D. Gynecological uses of hypnotism. In L. M. LeCron (Ed.), *Techniques of Hypnotherapy.* New York: Julian Press, 1961.

COUÉ, E. *Self-Mastery through Conscious Autosuggestion.* London: George Allen & Unwin, 1922.

COX, T. H. & ARAOZ, D. L. Sexual excitement and response by imagery production. *Journal of the American Society of Psychosomatic Dentistry & Medicine,* 1977, 23, 82-93.

CRASILNECK, H. B. & HALL, J. A. *Clinical Hypnosis: Principles and Applications.* New York: Grune & Stratton, 1975.

DeROPP, R. S. *Sex Energy.* New York: Delacorte Press, 1969.

DeSTEFANO, R. The "inoculation" effect in think-with instructions for "hypnotic-like" experiences. Unpublished doctoral dissertation, Temple University, 1977.

DEUTSCH, S. & SHERMAN, L. Impotence before diabetes. *Emergency Medicine.* 1981, 13, 7, 106.

DIAMOND, M. J. Modification of hypnotizability: A review. *Psychological Bulletin,* 1974, 81, 180-198.

DIAMOND, M. J. Hypnotizability is modifiable: An alternative approach. *International Journal of Clinical and Experimental Hypnosis,* 1977, 25, 147-166 (a).

DIAMOND, M. J. Issues and methods for modifying responsivity to hypnosis. *Annals of the N.Y. Academy of Sciences,* 1977, 269, 119-128 (b).

DIAMOND, M. J. *Clinical hypnosis: Toward a cognitive-based skill approach.* Paper presented at the 86th Annual Convention of the American Psychological Association. Toronto, August, 1978.

DIAMOND, M. J. The client-as-hypnotist: Furthering hypnotherapeutic change. *International Journal of Clinical Experimental Hypnosis,* 1980, 28, 197-207.

DITTBORN, J. Hypnotherapy of sexual impotence. *International Journal of Clinical and Experimental Hypnosis,* 1957, 5, 181-192.

DUBOIS, P. *The Psychic Treatment of Nervous Disorders: The Psychoneuroses and their Moral Treatment.* New York: Funk & Wagnalls, 1905.

EDELSTIEN, M. G. *Trauma, Trance and Transformation: A Clinical Guide to Hypnotherapy.* New York: Brunner/Mazel, 1981.

ELIADE, M. *Yoga: Immortality and Freedom.* New York: Pantheon, 1958.

ELLIS, A. *Reason and Emotion in Psychotherapy.* New York: Stuart, 1962.

ELLIS, A. *Sex Without Guilt.* New York: Lancer Books, 1966.

ELLIS, A. *Sex and the Liberated Man.* New York: Stuart, 1976.

ELLIS, A. & HARPER, R. A. *A Guide to Rational Living.* Englewood Cliffs, N.J.: Prentice-Hall, 1961.

ERICKSON, M. H. A study of an experimental neurosis hypnotically induced in a case of ejaculatio precox. *British Journal of Medical Psychology,* 1935, 15, 34-50.

ERICKSON, M. H. The interspersal hypnotic technique for symptom correction and pain control. *American Journal of Clinical Hypnosis,* 1966, 8, 198-209.

ERICKSON, M. H. & ROSSI, E. L. *Hypnotherapy: An Exploratory Casebook.* New York: Irvington, 1979.

EVANS, F. J. Hypnosis and sleep: Techniques for exploring cognitive activity during sleep. In E. Fromm & R. E. Shor (Eds.), *Hypnosis: Developments in Research and New Perspectives.* Chicago: Aldine, 1979.

EYSENCK, H. J. *Behaviour Therapy and the Neuroses.* Oxford: Pergamon, 1960.

EYSENCK, H. J. *Experiments in Behaviour Therapy.* Oxford: Pergamon, 1964.

EYSENCK, H. J. & EYSENCK, S. B. The validity of questionnaires and rating assessments of extraversion and neuroticism and their factorial validity. *British Journal of Psychology,* 1963, 54, 51-62.

FIELD, P. B. Humanistic aspects of hypnotic communication. In E. Fromm & R. E. Shor (Eds.), *Hypnosis: Developments in Research and New Perspectives.* New York: Aldine, 1969.

FISHER, S. *The Female Orgasm.* New York: Basic Books, 1973.

FISHMAN, S. T. & LUBETKIN, B. S. Maintenance and generalization of individual behavior therapy programs: clinical observations. In P. Karoly & J. J. Steffen (Eds.), *Improving the Long Term Effects of Psychotherapy.* New York: Gardner, 1980.

FLOWERS, J. V. & BOORAEM, C. D. Imagination training in the treatment of sexual dysfunction. *The Counseling Psychologist,* 1975, 5, 1, 50-51.

FRANKEL, F. H. *Hypnosis: Trance as a Coping Mechanism.* New York: Plenum, 1976.

FRANKS, C. M., & WILSON, G. T. *Annual Review of Behavior Therapy: Theory and Practice* (Vols. 1-7). New York: Brunner/Mazel. 1973-1979.

FREUD, S. Creative writers and daydreaming. In J. Strachey (Ed.), *The Standard Edition of the Complete Psychological Works of Sigmund Freud.* (Orig. publ., 1908) Vol. 9, London: Hogarth, 1962.

FROMM, E. An ego-psychological theory of altered states of consciousness. *The International Journal of Clinical and Experimental Hypnosis,* 1977, 25, 372-387.

FROMM, E. Values in hypnotherapy. *Psychotherapy: Theory, Research and Practice,* 1981, 17, 425-430.

FROMM, E., BROWN, D. P., HURT, S. W., OBERLANDER, J. Z., BOXER, A. M. & PFEIFER, G. The phenomena and characteristics of self-hypnosis. *International Journal of Clinical and Experimental Hypnosis,* 1981, 29, 189-246.

FROMM, E., OBERLANDER, M. I., & GRUENEWALD, D. Perceptual and cognitive processes in different states of consciousness: The waking state and hypnosis. *Journal of Projective Techniques and Personality Assessment,* 1970, 34, 375-387.

FROMME, A. *The Psychologist Looks at Sex and Marriage.* New York: Prentice-Hall, 1950.

GILBERT, S. F. Homosexuality and hypnotherapy. *British Journal of Medical Hypnosis,* 1954, 5, 2-11.

GOLDBERG, H. *The Hazards of Being Male.* New York: New American Library, 1976.

GOLDFRIED, M. R. Systematic desensitization as training in self-control. *Journal of Consulting and Clinical Psychology,* 1971, 37, 228-234.

GOLDMAN, M. H. Medical evaluation of sexually impotent men. *The Relationship,* 1981, 7, 6, 13.

GRAVITZ, M. A. & GERTON, M. I. Freud and Hypnosis: Report of post-rejection use. *Journal of the History of the Behavioral Sciences,* 1981, 17, 68-74.

HALEY, J. (Ed.). *Advanced Techniques of Hypnosis and Therapy: Selected Papers of M. H. Erickson.* New York: Grune & Stratton, 1967.

HARITON, E. B. The sexual fantasies of women. *Psychology Today,* March 1973, 39-44.

HARITON, E. B. & SINGER, J. L. Women's fantasies during sexual intercourse. *Journal of Consulting and Clinical Psychology,* 1974, 42, 313-322.

HARRIS, H., YULIS, S. & LACOSTE, D. Relationships among sexual arousability, imagery ability, and introversion-extraversion. *The Journal of Sex Research,* 1980, 16, 72-86.

HARTLAND, J. *Medical and Dental Hypnosis and Its Clinical Applications* (2nd ed.). Baltimore: Williams & Wilkins, 1975.

HASTINGS, D. W. *Impotence and Frigidity.* Boston: Little, Brown, 1963.

HAVENS, R. A. Contacting the "unconditioned other": Hypnosis as a mode of communication. *Voices,* 1981, 17, 1, 36-40.

HIATT, J. & KRIPKE, D. Ultradian rhythms in waking gastric activity. *Psychosomatic Medicine,* 1975, 37, 320-325.

HILGARD, E. R. *Hypnotic Susceptibility.* New York: Harcourt, Brace & World, 1965.

HILGARD, E. R. The problem of divided consciousness: A neodissociation interpretation. *Annals of the N.Y. Academy of Sciences,* 1977, 296, 48-59 (a).

HILGARD, E. R. *Divided Consciousness: Multiple Controls in Human Thought and Action.* New York: Wiley-Interscience, 1977 (b).

HILGARD, E. R. & HILGARD, J. R. *Hypnosis in the Relief of Pain.* Los Altos, CA.: Wm. Kaufman, Inc., 1975.

HILGARD, J. R. *Personality and Hypnosis: A Study of Imaginative Involvement.* Chicago: The University of Chicago Press, 1970.

HILL, N. *Think and Be Rich.* North Hollywood, CA.: Wilshire, 1966.

HOGAN, D. R. The Effectiveness of Sex Therapy: A review of the literature. In LoPiccolo, J. & LoPiccolo, L. (Eds.), *Handbook of Sex Therapy.* New York: Plenum, 1978.

HOLLENDER, M. H. Women's fantasies during sexual intercourse. *Archives of General Psychiatry,* 1963, 8, 86-90.

HOON, E. F., HOON, P. W. & WINCZE, J. P. An inventory for the measurement of female sexual arousability: The SAI. *Archives of Sexual Behavior,* 1976, 5, 291-300.

HULL, C. L. *Hypnosis and Suggestibility.* New York: Appleton-Century, 1933.

HUSSAIN, A. Behavior therapy using hypnosis. In J. Wolpe, A. Solter & L. Reyna (Eds.), *The Conditioning Therapies: The Challenge in Psychotherapy.* New York: Rinehart & Winston, 1964.

JANDA, L. H. & O'GRADY, K. E. Development of a sex anxiety inventory. *Journal of Consulting and Clinical Psychology,* 1980, 48, 169-175.

JEHU, D. *Sexual Dysfunction.* New York: John Wiley & Sons, 1979.

KAPLAN, H. S. *The New Sex Therapy.* New York: Brunner/Mazel, 1974.

KAPLAN, H. S. *The Illustrated Manual of Sex Therapy.* New York: New York Times Book Co., 1975.

KAPLAN, H. S. *Disorders of Sexual Desire.* New York: Brunner/Mazel, 1979.

KASSORLA, I. *Nice Girls Do—And Now You Can Too!* Los Angeles: Stratford Press, 1980.

KATZ, N. W. *Hypnotic inductions as training in self-control.* Paper presented at the 85th Annual Convention of the American Psychological Association, San Francisco, August, 1977.

KATZ, N. W. Hypnotic inductions as training in cognitive self-control. *Cognitive Therapy and Research,* 1978, 2, 365-369.

KATZ, N. W. Increasing hypnotic responsiveness: Behavioral training vs. trance induction. *Journal of Consulting and Clinical Psychology,* 1979, 47, 119-127.

KATZ, N. W. & CRAWFORD, V. L. *A little trance and a little skill: Interaction between models of hypnosis and type of hypnotic induction.* Paper presented at annual meeting of the Society for Clinical & Experimental Hypnosis, Ashville, N.C., October, 1978.

KAZDIN, A. E. Effects of covert modeling and modeling reinforcement on assertive behavior. *Journal of Abnormal Psychology,* 1974, 83, 240-252.

KIEFER, O. *Sexual Life in Ancient Rome.* London: Routledge and Kegan Paul, 1932.

KINNEY, J. M. & SACHS, L. B. Increasing hypnotic susceptibility. *Journal of Abnormal Psychology,* 1974, 83, 145-150.

KINSEY, A. C., POMEROY, W. B., MARTIN, C. E. & GEBHARD, P. H. *Sexual Behavior in the Human Female.* Philadelphia: Saunders, 1953.

KORZYBSKI, A. *Science and Sanity,* (4th Ed.). Lakeville, CT: The International Non-Aristotelian Library Publishing Co., 1933.

KRIS, E. *Psychoanalytic Explorations in Art.* New York: International Universities Press, 1952 (Orig. publ. 1934).

KRIS, E. The recovery of childhood memories. *The Psychoanalytical Study of the Child.* 1956, 11, 54-88.

KROGER, W. *Clinical and Experimental Hypnosis* (2nd edition). Philadelphia: Lippincott, 1977.

KROGER, W. S. & ALLE, J. E. Paradise regained: Liberating sexually inhibited patients through hypnotic behavioral conditioning. *Behavioral Medicine,* 1981, 8, 9, 13-21.

KROGER, W. S. & FEZLER, W. D. *Hypnosis and Behavior Modification: Imagery Conditioning.* Philadelphia: Lippincott, 1976.

LAZARUS, A. A. *Behavior Therapy and Beyond.* New York: McGraw-Hill, 1971.

LAZARUS, A. A. "Hypnosis" as a facilitator in behavior therapy. *International Journal of Clinical and Experimental Hypnosis,* 1973, 21, 25-31.

LAZARUS, A. A. *Multimodal Behavior Therapy.* New York: Springer, 1976.

LAZARUS, A. A. *In the Mind's Eye.* New York: Rawson, 1977.

LECKIE, F. H. Hypnotherapy in gynecological disorders. *International Journal of Clinical and Experimental Hypnosis.* 1964, 12, 121-146.

LERMAN, H. Review of *Frigidity,* by G. S. Macvaugh. *Journal of Sex Research,* 1980, 16, 1, 87-88.

LESHAN, L. *You Can Fight for Your Life.* New York: Harcourt Brace Jovanovich, 1977.

LICHT, H. *Sexual Life in Ancient Greece.* London: Brandt, 1932.

LIEBERMAN, L. R. Hypnosis research and the limitations of the experimental method. *Annals of the New York Academy of Sciences,* 1977, 296, 60-68.

LIEF, H. I. Inhibited sexual desire. *Medical Aspects of Human Sexuality,* 1977, 11, 7, 94-95.

LoPICCOLO, J. The professionalization of sex therapy: Issues and problems. In J. LoPiccolo & L. LoPiccolo (Eds.), *Handbook of Sex Therapy.* New York: Plenum, 1978.

LoPICCOLO, J, & LoPICCOLO, L. (Eds.). *Handbook of Sex Therapy.* New York: Plenum, 1978.

LoPICCOLO, L. Low Sexual Desire. In S. R. Leiblum and L. A. Pervin (Eds.). *Principles and Practice of Sex Therapy.* New York: Guilford, 1980.

LOZANOV, G. *Suggestology and Outlines of Suggestology.* New York: Gordon & Breach, 1978.

LURIA, A. *The Role of Speech in the Regulation of Normal and Abnormal Behavior.* New York: Liveright, 1961.

LUTZKER, D. R. Treating medical patients with hypnosis. *Nassau County Medical Center Proceedings,* Winter, 1981, 26-29.

MACVOUGH, G. S. *Frigidity: What You Should Know about Its Cure with Hypnosis.* Elmsford, N.Y.: Pergamon, 1979.

MALTZ, M. *Psycho-cybernetics.* New York: Prentice-Hall, 1960.

MARTIN, P. A. The happy sexless marriage. *Medical Aspects of Human Sexuality,* 1977, 11, 5, 75-85.

MASTERS, W. H. & JOHNSON, V. E. *Human Sexual Response.* Boston: Little, Brown, 1966.

MASTERS, W. H. & JOHNSON, V. E. *Human Sexual Inadequacy.* Boston: Little, Brown, 1970.

MASTERS, W. H. & JOHNSON, V. E. *Homosexuality in Perspective.* Boston: Little, Brown, 1979.

MEICHENBAUM, D. Cognitive factors in behavior modification: Modifying what clients say to themselves. In C. M. Franks & G. T. Wilson, (Eds.). *Annual Review of Behavior Therapy: Theory and Practice* (Vol. 1). New York: Brunner/Mazel, 1973.

MEICHENBAUM, D. *Cognitive Behavior Modification.* Morristown, N.J.: General Learning Press, 1974.

MEICHENBAUM, D. *Cognitive Behavior Modification.* New York: Plenum, 1977.

MEICHENBAUM, D. Why does using imagery in psychotherapy lead to change? In J. L. Singer & K. S. Pope (Eds.), *The Power of Human Imagination.* New York: Plenum, 1978 (a).

MEICHENBAUM, D. Introduction to applied cognitive behavior therapy. In D. Meichenbaum, (Ed.), *Cognitive Behavior Therapy: A Practitioner's Guide.* New York: B.M.A. Audio Cassettes, 1978 (b).

MEICHENBAUM, D. & CAMERON, R. Training schizophrenics to talk to themselves: A means of developing attentional controls. *Behavior Therapy,* 1973, 4, 515-534.

MITCHELL, K. M., BOZARTH, J. D. & KRAUFT, C. C. A re-appraisal of the therapeutic effectiveness of accurate empathy, nonpossessive warmth and genuineness. In A. S. Gurman & A. M. Razin (Eds.), *Effective Psychotherapy: A Handbook of Research.* New York: Pergamon, 1977.

MONTAGU, A. *Touching: The Human Significance of the Skin.* New York: Harper & Row, 1978.

MOSHER, D. L. Interaction of fear and guilt in inhibiting unacceptable behavior. *Journal of Con-*

sulting Psychology, 1965, 29, 161-167.

MOSHER, D. L. The development and multitrait-multimethod matrix analysis of three measures of three aspects of guilt. *Journal of Consulting Psychology*, 1966, 30, 25-29.

MOSHER, D. L. Three dimensions of depth of involvement in human sexual response. *Journal of Sex Research*, 1980, 16, 1-42.

MOSHER, D. L. & WHITE, B. B. Effects of committed or casual erotic guided imagery on females' subjective sexual arousal and emotional response. *The Journal of Sex Research*, 1980, 16, 273-299.

NIDEFFER, R. M. *The Inner Athlete*. New York: Crowell, 1976.

ORNE, M. T. The construct of hypnosis: Implications of the definition for research and practice. *Annals of the New York Academy of Sciences*, 1977, 296, 14-33.

PAVIO, A. Mental imagery, associative learning and memory. *Psychological Review*, 1969, 76, 241-263.

PELLETIER, A. M. Three uses of guided imagery in hypnosis. *American Journal of Clinical Hypnosis*, 1979, 22, 32-36.

PELLETIER, K. R. *Holistic Medicine*. New York: Delacorte Press, 1979.

PERLS, F. S. *Gestalt Therapy Verbatim*. Ed. by J. Stevens. Lafayette, CA.: Real People Press, 1969.

PIETROPINTO, A. & SIMENAUER, J. *Beyond the Male Myth: What Women Want to Know about Men's Sexuality*. New York: Times Books, 1977.

PLATONOV, K. *The Word as a Physiological and Therapeutic Factor*. Moscow: Foreign Language Publishing House, 1959.

RAHULA, W. S. *What the Buddha Taught*. London: Gordon Frazer, 1959.

RALEY, P. E. *Making Love*. New York: Dial Press, 1976.

RAPAPORT, D. States of consciousness: A psychopathological and psychodynamic view. In M. M. Gill (Ed.), *The Collected Papers of David Rapaport*. New York: Basic Books, 1967.

REILLEY, R. R., PERISHER, D. W., CORONA, A. & DOBROVOLSKY, N. W. Modifying hypnotic susceptibility by practice and instruction. *International Journal of Clinical and Experimental Hypnosis*, 1980, 28, 39-45.

ROMANCZYK, R. G. & KISTNER, J. J. The current state of the arts in behavior modification. *The Psychotherapy Bulletin*, 1977, 11, 4, 16-30.

ROSEN, R. C., LEIBLUM, S. R. & GAGNON, J. H. *Sexual scripts, assessment and modification in sex therapy*. Paper presented at the fifth annual meeting of the Society for Sex Therapy and Research, Philadelphia, March, 1979.

SACERDOTE, P. *Induced Dreams*. New York: Vantage, 1967.

SACHS, L. B. & ANDERSON, W. L. Modification of hypnotic susceptibility. *International Journal of Clinical & Experimental Hypnosis*, 1967, 15, 172-180.

SANDERS, S. Mutual group hypnosis as a catalyst in fostering creative problem solving. *American Journal of Clinical Hypnosis*, 1976, 19, 62-66.

SARBIN, T. R. Contributions to role-taking theory: I. Hypnotic behavior. *Psychological review*, 1950, 57, 255-270.

SARBIN, T. R. & COE, W. C. *Hypnosis: A Social Psychological Analysis of Influence Communication*. New York: Rinehart & Winston, 1972.

SCHNECK, J. M. Hypnotherapy for vaginismus. *International Journal of Clinical and Experimental Hypnosis*, 1965, 13, 92-95.

SHAMES, R. & STERIN, C. *Healing with Mind Power*. Emmaus, PA.: Rodale Press, 1978.

SHARPE, R. & MEYER, V. Modification of "cognitive sexual pain" by the spouse under supervision. *Behavior Therapy*, 1973, 4, 285-287.

SHEEHAN, P. W. A shortened form of Bett's questionnaire upon Mental Imagery. *Journal of Clinical Psychology*, 1967, 23, 286-289.

SHEEHAN, P. W. Imagery process and hypnosis: An experiential analysis of phenomena. In A. A. Sheikh & J. T. Shaffer (Eds.), *The Potential of Human Fantasy and Imagination*.

New York: Brandon House, 1979.

SHEIKH, A. A. & SHAFFER, J. T. (Eds.). *The Potential of Fantasy and Imagination*. New York: Brandon House, 1979.

SHOR, R. E. & ORNE, E. C. *Harvard Group Scale of Hypnotic Susceptibility*. Palo Alto, CA.: Consulting Psychologists Press, 1962.

SHORR, J. *Psychotherapy Through Imagery*. New York: Intercontinental Medical Corp., 1974.

SHORR, J. *Go See the Movie in Your Head*. New York: Popular Library, 1977.

SINGER, J. L. *The Inner World of Daydreaming*. New York: Harper & Row, 1975.

SINGER, J. L. Imagery and affect in psychotherapy: Elaborating private scripts and generating contexts. In A. A. Sheikh & J. T. Shaffer (Eds.), *The Potential of Fantasy and Imagination*. New York: Brandon House, 1979.

SINGER, J. L. & McCRAVEN, V. Some characteristics of adult daydreaming. *Journal of Psychology*, 1961, 51, 151-164.

SINGER, J. L. & POPE, K. S. (Eds.). *The Power of Human Imagination*. New York: Plenum, 1978.

SINGER, J. L. & POPE, K. S. Daydreaming and Imagery skills as predisposing capacities for self-hypnosis. *International Journal of Clinical and Experimental Hypnosis*, 1981, 29, 271-281.

SKINNER, B. F. *Science and Human Behavior*. New York: Macmillan, 1953.

SKINNER, B. F. *Beyond Freedom and Dignity*. New York: Knopf, 1971.

SPANOS, N. P. Goal-directed fantasy and the performance of hypnotic test suggestions. *Psychiatry*, 1971, 34, 86-96.

SPANOS, N. P. & BARBER, T. X. Cognitive activity during "hypnotic" suggestibility: goal-directed fantasy and the experience of non-volition. *Journal of Personality*, 1972, 40, 510-524.

SPRINGER, K. J. Effectiveness of Treatment of Sexual Dysfunction: Review and Evaluation. *Journal of Sex Education and Therapy*, 1981, 7, 1, 18-22.

STAAS, A. W. Language behavior therapy: A derivative of social behaviorism. *Behavior Therapy*, 1972, 2, 165-192.

STEGER, J. C. Cognitive behavior strategies in the treatment of sexual problems. In J. P. Foreyt & D. P. Rathjen (Eds.), *Cognitive Behavior Therapy*, New York: Plenum, 1978.

SUINN, R. M. & RICHARDSON, F. Anxiety management training: A non-specific behavior therapy program for anxiety control. *Behavior Therapy*, 1971, 2, 498-510.

TANNAHILL, R. *Sex in History*. New York: Stein & Day, 1980.

TART, C. T. Quick and convenient assessment of hypnotic depth: Self-report scales. *American Journal of Clinical Hypnosis*, 1979, 21, 186-207.

TAYLOR, G. R. *Sex in History*. New York: Vanguard Press, 1954.

The Counseling Psychologist. Sex Counseling, 1975, 5, 1.

TILTON, P. *Personal Communication*, February, 1981.

TRUAX, C. B. & CARKHUFF, R. R. *Towards Effective Counseling and Psychotherapy: Training and Practice*. Chicago: Aldine, 1967.

TUGENDER, H. S. & FERINDEN, W. E. *An Introduction to Hypno-Operant Therapy*. Orange, N.J.: Power Publishers, 1972.

VAN PELT, S. J. *Hypnotism and its importance in medicine*. Paper presented at University College, London, May, 1949.

VAN PELT, S. J. *Secrets of Hypnotism*. North Hollywood, CA., 1958 (New edition, 1974).

WALEN, S. R. Cognitive factors in sexual behavior. *Journal of Sex and Marital Therapy*, 1980, 6, 87-101.

WALEN, S. R. Personal communication, January 13, 1981.

WATKINS, J. *The Therapeutic Self*. New York: Human Sciences Press, 1978.

WATZLAWICK, P. *The Language of Change*. New York: Basic Books, 1978.

WEAR, J. B. Causes of dyspareunia in men. *Medical Aspects of Human Sexuality*, 1976, 10, 5, 140-153.

WEITZENHOFFER, A. M. *General Techniques of Hypnotism.* New York: Grune & Stratton, 1957.

WEITZENHOFFER, A. M. Hypnotic susceptibility revisited. *American Journal of Clinical Hypnosis,* 1980, 22, 130-146.

WEITZENHOFFER, A. M. & HILGARD, E. R. *Stanford Hypnotic Susceptibility Scale, Forms A and B.* Palo Alto, CA.: Consulting Psychologists Press, 1959.

WEITZENHOFFER, A. M. & HILGARD, E. R. *Stanford Hypnotic Susceptibility Scale, Form C,* Palo Alto, CA.: Consulting Psychologists Press, 1962.

WICK, E. The Hypnotic State as a Receptive State. Unpublished manuscript, St. John's University, 1981.

WILKINS, W. Parameters of therapeutic imagery: Directions from case studies. *Psychotherapy: Theory, Research and Practice,* 1974, 11, 163-171.

WILSON, G. T. Cognitive behavior therapy: Paradigm shift or passing phase? In J. P. Foreyt & D. P. Rathjen (Eds.), *Cognitive Behavior Therapy: Research and Application,* New York: Plenum, 1978 (a).

WILSON, G. T. *Cognitive Behavioral Approaches to Sexual Problems.* B.M.A. Audio Cassettes. New York: Guilford Publications, Inc. 1978 (b).

WINOKUR, G. & LEONARD, C. Sexual life in patients with hysteria. *Diseases of the Nervous System,* 1963, 24, 337-342.

WISH, P. A. The use of imagery-based techniques in the treatment of sexual dysfunction. *The Counseling Psychologist,* 1975, 5, 1, 52-55.

WOLBERG, L. R. *Hypnoanalysis.* New York: Grune & Stratton, 1945 (Second ed. 1964).

WOLFE, L. *The Cosmo Report.* New York: Arbor House, 1981.

WOLLMAN, L. *Sexual disorders managed by hypnotherapy.* Paper presented at the meeting of the Society for the Scientific Study of Sex, January 10, 1964.

WOLPE, J. *Psychotherapy by Reciprocal Inhibition.* Stanford: Stanford University Press, 1958.

WOLPIN, M. Guided imagining to reduce avoidance behavior. *Psychotherapy: Theory, Research and Practice,* 1969, 6, 122-124.

ZILBERGELD, B. *Male Sexuality.* Boston: Little, Brown, 1978.

ZILBERGELD, B. & EVANS, M. The inadequacy of Masters and Johnson. *Psychology Today,* Aug. 1980, 14, 3, 128-43.

Index

171